D0822125

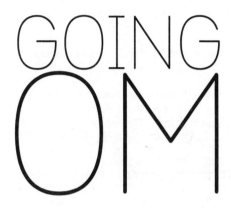

GOING OM

Real-Life Stories On
and Off the Yoga Mat

EDITED BY
Melissa Carroll

FOREWORD BY
Cheryl Strayed

viva
EDITIONS

Published in the United States by Viva Editions, an imprint of Cleis Press, Inc., 2246 Sixth Street, Berkeley, California 94710.

Printed in the United States.
Cover design: Scott Idleman/Blink
Cover photograph: Joshua Hodge Photography/Getty Images
Text design: Frank Wiedemann

First Edition.
10 9 8 7 6 5 4 3 2 1

Trade paper ISBN: 978-1-936740-86-4
E-book ISBN: 978-1-936740-98-7

Library of Congress Cataloging-in-Publication Data

Going Om : real-life stories on and off the yoga mat / edited by Melissa Carroll.
    pages cm
    ISBN 978-1-936740-86-4 (paperback) -- ISBN 978-1-936740-98-7 (ebook)
    1. Mind and body. 2. Yoga. I. Carroll, Melissa.
    BF161.G56 2014
    613.7'0460922--dc23
                                2014007101

Welcome OM

We unroll a mat and, unexpectedly, we fall in love. We fall in love with the way we can feel in these moving, breathing bodies of ours. We fall in love with the sweetness of stillness. As Lisa Knopp says in her tender essay, "I hadn't expected to be transformed by yoga." And yet we are. We continue to be transformed, time and time again. This constant shifting, of course, permeates beyond the incense-laced yoga studios, touching all facets of our lives.

Which is probably why if you say you practice yoga in 2014, more than 20 million Americans will nod and grin, having also wiggled through a Sun Salutation. But if you said the word *yoga* fifty years ago at the workplace or a dinner party, you may as well have just claimed to sacrifice toddlers in the name of Lord Vishnu. Yoga seeped into the United States from India in 1900, but it took nearly the entire century for the practice to carve its way into the country's cultural and emotional landscape.

And now its popularity is undeniable: from Key West to Prudhoe Bay, yoga studios have cropped up in strip malls and small towns, next to pizzerias and karate dojos. Yoga got trendy, hippie turned hot, Buddha became badass. Yoga pants are the new jeans.

We know yoga has assimilated into the American mainstream, from Power Fusion to Naked Yoga to Doga: Yoga with Your Dog. But what draws millions of Americans to the mat? How has the pulse of our lives pushed us to touch the center of stillness? What exactly are we searching for? And what do we find once we get there?

Going OM is an exploration of these questions, through candid, witty, and courageous literary nonfiction.

When compiling the essays for this book, I wanted to capture the real experiences of "regular" people on and off the mat. Not rubber bands, not Cirque du Soleil extras, not wisdom-spouting sages. As Neal Pollack opens his essay: "When you think of a 'yogi,' my dad isn't what comes to mind, unless you're thinking of Yogi Bear." I didn't ask yoga masters to contribute; I asked writers.

Just as yoga and meditation are paths within, writing is a path to better understand ourselves and the world around us. To write is to translate the world. To be a writer or a yogi, we must be observers. We must quietly witness and patiently absorb all the wonder, seeming confusion, and paradoxical beauty that exists. Both writers and yoga students seek to make meaning of this wildly miraculous human experience.

I was more interested in the stories of people who can't touch their toes, who have known loss, who have felt deeply insecure in the back row of a class, sweating while seeking a little self-love. Some of the finest national bestselling and up-and-coming writers have shared their stories, their insights, and their lives in this book: what emerged has blown me away.

What bubbled up again and again in so many of these essays? Struggle, self-doubt, relationships, the frenetic brain with its *to-do lists* and *what-ifs* and *I'm-not-good-enoughs*. How, for most of us mere mortals, our bodies are not the sinewy, Lululemon-clad acrobats posing in yoga magazines. And we are stunning in our imperfections, though that term doesn't feel right—perhaps *humanness* is more appropriate. We are stunning in our humanness, and in many of these brilliant, touching, hilarious essays, the practice of yoga—with its stumbling and flailing and unfolding—reveals our humanness to ourselves.

Claire Dederer so astutely says in her essay, "We all have a deep need to be in our bodies, experiencing them with immediacy. Unhindered by the patterning of consciousness."

Throughout *Going OM*, the body is encountered again and again, in its myriad forms and manifestations. Ira Sukrungruang's deeply moving "Body Replies" recounts his relationship with his four-hundred-pound diabetic body, his yoga, and his self-image. Emily Rapp pulls back the veil of the self in an Ashtanga class—as a woman with an artificial leg who is a former anorexic, she reveals that ultimately what we are seeking is not technical perfection but acceptance and aliveness: to be seen for precisely who we are and to know that, yes, we can be enough.

The writers of *Going OM* have felt the heft of loss drop them heavier into the earth. They have been made vulnerable because life has broken them open. But there is openness in the breaking places. Those openings offer space for the breath to move. And breath, not surprisingly, is a theme we return to again and again.

In yoga we are taught how to breathe, something we've done our entire lives, and yet something we don't usually do well. With equal parts tenderness and humor, Suzanne Morrison weaves the narrative of her mother's breast cancer with her own struggle gasping for air in her life, and how she learned, through cigarettes, singing, and *pranayama*, to breathe a little easier. Sonya Huber depicts her similar quest to take a deep breath: as she puts it, "My throat chakra is all jacked up." Adriana Páramo tells her gripping narrative of betrayal, redemption, and love, when she locks herself in a British mansion during her stepdaughter's elegant wedding and then employs Eastern philosophy to ease a panic attack. Dani Shapiro's keen awareness of "the all of it"—the richness in both the mundane and the meaningful—helps us recognize the preciousness of the present.

We know yoga is so much richer than just a series of poses, though the physicality of the practice often opens us up to the deeper, metaphoric, and more spiritual elements. With incandescent wit and wisdom, Claire Dederer candidly talks about yoga's inherent sexiness (there certainly is a lot of bending over in tight pants), which is really about our inhabiting this body of ours. Jason Tucker links his father's lifetime labor as a machinist in rural Alabama to yogic insights. Plus, in two essays, dogs are the teachers, helping authors Brenda Miller and Adriana Páramo remember the fullness of the present. (I've always said dogs were natural yoga masters. We modeled one of the most recognizable postures after them!)

Going OM connects these vibrant, diverse voices to bridge the individual experience of yoga with the collective. The very act of writing is an act of connection, and in this we are reminded that we are not, in fact, alone.

Reading these heart-wrenching and yet often hilarious stories reminded me of my first yoga class in 2006. I was twenty-two and, like so many, wanted to find meaning in my life. And like so many, I searched for it in the external: I was grasping for happiness in objects, in other people, and in my ideas about who I should be. The religion I had grown up with left me questioning, and nights of partying left me unfulfilled. I'd wrestled with depression, anxiety, and chronic headaches since I was nine. There was this knot of sadness lodged deep within me—it felt at once acute and vague—and I had no idea how it got there. I wanted to feel at ease in my own skin, not tossed by the changing winds of circumstance. I wanted what I think ultimately everyone wants: a little slice of inner peace.

My local yoga studio in Tampa offered a free beginner class. Feeling awkward in my spandex pants, I borrowed a mat and unrolled it in the back row. Inside, tea lights glinted from the hardwood floor while soft instrumental music played from a stereo.

The instructor, a tall woman with long hair, spoke softly: "Drink in a breath and close your eyes. I invite you to let go of your notions about your body, what you should look like, how you think you should move. However you look, however you are, is perfect in this moment."

Suddenly tears singed my eyes. I usually cried when something felt right. My body slowly uncoiled. I stretched curiously like a newborn, unpeeling the tightness within me. After class, for what seemed like the first time, my mind felt clear and open. I was content. Not necessarily happy, because contentment lasts longer than happiness. Contentment comes from within. It doesn't depend on the new car, the promotion at work, or the lover's attention to exist. It exists simply because it can. Who cared if I couldn't touch my toes? I knew from that very first class that I was going to teach this yoga stuff.

Enlightenment, of course, is not instant. I'm a slow learner.

But I see how the practice of gratitude has helped keep me content amid the tides. Yoga and meditation have helped me cope when life has changed on me unexpectedly, as life is wont to do. I have been teaching yoga now for more than six years, and still have a lot to learn. But this is precisely why yoga is called a practice. It takes a whole lifetime (and if you're into reincarnation, a few thousand lifetimes), and it is in this journey, this practice, that we come to realize the fullness of our lives. To find some meaning, whatever path or shape that takes. And ultimately, to love.

It is often said that yoga is a coming home; back to our true selves, underneath the layers of busy thoughts, waves of emotions, and clenched muscles. With that spirit I cheer you on your journey home to yourself, your journey back to love. May these stories inspire you, delight you, and move you, as they have for me. Thank you for *Going OM*.

Cheers & *namaste*,
Melissa Carroll, Editor
June 2013

Lokah samastah sukhino bhavantu
May all beings everywhere be happy and free

Contents

Foreword

Cheryl Strayed

The first time I found myself on a yoga mat I was three years old, enrolled in a class at a YMCA in Pittsburgh. We made mountains with our arms and triangles with our legs. "Here's something you can do when you watch TV!" the teacher exclaimed in a sing-song voice as she wound her limbs into what I'd later know to be Sitting Eagle pose. I twisted myself into a rough imitation of her and felt that lovely, tingly burn that nothing else quite replicates. So began my lifelong love affair with yoga.

It's been a complicated relationship. In some eras of my life, yoga has been a mainstay of my week. I've done yoga in Portland and New York and Minnesota, in Thailand and Costa Rica, in hot rooms, on windy balconies and with my infant children cradled in my arms. In other eras, entire seasons glided past without my having once attempted to touch my toes, let alone held myself in a Warrior pose. And yet even in the times when I'm not doing it, yoga is always there for me, a presence in my body even when it's not actually in my daily life. It's the thing I do when I'm doing everything right; the thing I intend to return to doing when I've gotten off track. Yoga is part of the life I most deeply want to live even if I'm not currently living it.

My struggle toward a consistent dose of *om* in my life goes
beyond yoga, of course. I think that's what's so compelling about yoga
to me. It isn't about how to work out, but how to *be*. And when it
comes to that, like most of us, I'm a work in progress. I was reminded
of that in a yoga class a few years ago in which the teacher often
lectured us on the importance of Savasana—the so-called "corpse"
pose one gets to do at the end of class. It was the one pose I thought
I could master since it seemingly required nothing aside from lying
there taking a half-nap. But no. After he'd led us through a comically
impossible series of twists and bends and stretches, it was this pose—
the one that seemed the simplest of all—that was actually the most
difficult to do, he asserted. In Savasana, he explained, your work is
to not work. Your task is to surrender to the strange reality of having
no task, to allow awareness to fall away into nothing but the breath.
Breathing in. Breathing out. To play dead while never feeling quite so
spectacularly alive.

Perhaps that's the reason I admire the essays in this collection
so deeply. Like Savasana, they seem to be one thing—writers on the
subject of yoga—but really they're another: profound examinations of
what it means to be human. In this collection, there are funny stories,
sad stories, moving stories, and real stories. In sharing their experiences with us, each of these writers have tapped into the universal
questions that we're confronted with when we get ourselves down on
the mat. Questions about humility and determination. Simplicity and
acceptance. About moving forward, doing the work, and most of all,
receiving with equanimity what comes next one breath at a time.

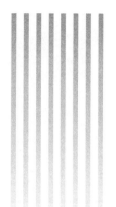

PART ONE

BREATHE

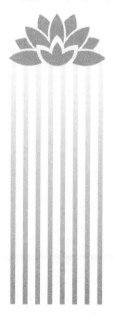

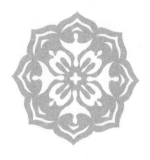

Ira Sukrungruang

Body Replies

*Our own physical body possesses a wisdom which we who
inhabit the body lack. We give it orders which make no
sense.*

—HENRY MILLER

Outside, winter rages. Snow blinds. White out conditions. The
wind is a guttural animal against this old upstate building. I
swear I feel the sway of this place, feel the cold invading the fissures of
the structure. I know after this session I will have to put on my heavy
boots and double-thick coat and enter the storm. I know I will have to
scrape and rescrape the snow and ice and slush off my car. And I know

that every warm muscle I have worked hard to stretch will shrink and tighten as soon as I step foot outside. Yet, right now, I'm here. My three-hundred-seventy-pound Body, occupying this space that is free of judgment, free of ridicule, free of self-loathing.

Mostly.

Peace pervades this yoga studio in Oswego, NY. Incense permeates the space—fragrant and earthy. Candles flicker on windowsill ledges, casting wavering light onto the wooden floors. Buddha presides in the front of the rectangular room. Over speakers is the sound of bells, like the ones tinkling on temples in Thailand.

Today, I am learning to walk.

We go from one end of the studio to the other, twelve of us in varying speeds and strides. Our instructor, Howard, tells us to feel the floor. "You are connected," he says.

I usually bristle at what sounds like New Age instruction, bristle at anything touchy-feely. Such sayings have struck me as melodramatic and unnecessarily deep—bad fortune cookie fortunes. But I let Howard's words sink in because I like Howard. I like his patience with me and Body, like his words of encouragement when I do positions Body is unaccustomed to. Plus, his gray beard is glorious.

I fixate on the word *connected*. I try to merge Body and mind. I say, step. I say, walk. I say, gentle. The opposite happens. My feet slap the floor, startling my glassy-eyed neighbor, who flinches at the sound. The floor creaks and cracks. I am painfully aware of how clumsy Body is, and when that happens I turn on myself. I say, fat. I say, ugly. I say, stupid.

"Walking is difficult," Howard says. "We never think about it. We are always doing."

4

I take another step. Slow. Concentrate. Lift the foot. Place pad of foot on floor. Follow with heel. Shift weight forward. Again.

"This is how we were meant to walk," Howard says. "No shoes. No socks. Skin against earth. Feel it. Let that sensation spread from the bottom of your body to the top."

I lose my balance. I stagger. I sigh.

"It's okay, Ira," Howard says. He moves behind me. Watches my steps.

Sweat drips from my forehead.

"You're walking on the outside of your feet," Howard says. "Make sure the whole bottom touches. Even the little toe."

I'm conscious of my loud walking, of my audible breaths, thick and hot. The others are like stealthy ninjas, gliding over the surface of the floor, absent of thought, just doing.

"What are you thinking?" Howard says.

I don't tell him the truth. I don't tell him how much I hate myself, how much I hate Body. I don't tell him how much I hate that I can't walk correctly.

"I'm thinking heel then toe," I say.

Howard doesn't buy it. He tilts his head and puts a hand to his bearded chin. It is the look Santa might give when he's deciphering whether you've been naughty or nice. "It seems you are disconnecting. Am I right?"

I shrug, but he is. My mind and Body are not one. Have never been one. They are separate entities. I have disconnected from Body, allowed it to do what it wants, when it wants. I have lost control. I started yoga to get it back. To connect to it. But this exercise of walking—fucking walking—has depleted hope that this will ever happen.

"You can do it," Howard says. "Give it time."

Being large and diabetic, time is something I may have little of.

❀ ❀ ❀

Body as language: You are a fat run-on sentence that feeds like high-schoolers on riblet day—no—hyenas at the feast—no—the famished and you are never sated never happy because you have long since forgotten what happiness feels like—real happiness—not the quick illusion of it every time you sit and eat because that happiness is temporary and what follows is a loathing that makes you want to pluck the hairs off your legs one at a time—no—scream until the throat bleeds—no—tear hunks of your meaty flesh and fling them off because when you eat you have forgotten the sensation of satisfaction the meaning of the word *enough* or *plenty* or *sufficient* or *full* because the word *full* suggests there is no more space no more room to justify one more bite of something that will cut your life by another year but the surprising thing is you find more room because there is always more to choke a heart to choke the veins to choke the arteries and still you can't help but feel that there are places in you that are empty and starving and you can't seem to feed them the right food can't seem to figure out this puzzle of hunger and you feel this endeavor is point-less like feeding goldfish pieces of goldfish—no—like a food critic at McDonald's—no—like a milk shake without the shake or the milk and these moments have become the saddest recognition of your life because it means you are powerless against what hurts you most which means you are powerless against your own self which means you can't stop what is sure to happen—who can?

楽 楽 楽

At the yoga studio, my favorite time is the darkness at the end, after we have worked out every muscle, after we have sweated and strained. Howard turns off the lights and we get into our relaxed positions—lying supine, legs raised on a chair—and concentrate on breathing. His voice leads us into our relaxed states.

"Close your eyes," Howard says, "and release all your worries."

The darkness is a comfort. It is a body pillow I cling to. In the light, Body is front and center. In the dark, it disappears. It ceases to matter.

"Relax your shoulders, your neck, your back," Howard says. "Chase away that tension with your breath."

I spend most of my day trying to disappear. Trying to squash Body. I have, in many ways, created a perpetual darkness in my life. Many fat people do this. To hide ourselves, we exaggerate another part of our personalities. I put on a wide smile. I nod voraciously. I ask questions. I make people laugh. In this way, I place persona in front of Body. I make people see someone else entirely. This, perhaps, is why fat people have been stereotyped as jolly or good-natured, why fat people are expected to smile and tell a joke. What people forget, however, is this is a mask. We deny ourselves true feeling; we belittle our suffering. What people forget is that it takes a lot of energy to wear this mask day in and day out. Yet, at the same time, we live in the darkness because we fear what would happen when we let the light in. We fear what we might discover. Worse yet, what others might discover.

"Imagine your stresses as paper," Howard says. "Crumple them up. Throw them away."

Darkness hides our flaws—yes—but it hides us, too. It is the reason the boys in my neighborhood loved playing hide-and-seek at night. Darkness provided extra cover. Darkness provided shadows. If you wore black, you could disappear entirely. One of us would never be found because he hid so well. We'd call his name. We'd say the game was over. We'd say it was time to go home before we got in trouble. And out came the best hider. He would emerge—usually climbing down the tallest tree or crawling out from underneath a Dumpster—and we would register his physicalness. First the outline of his body. Then his individual parts, the fingers, the feet. Then finally his face. His smile. He would be found. He would be part of this world again.

"Breathe deeply," Howard says. "Allow yourself to be only here, in this space."

I would have remained hidden. I would have stayed in my hiding spot for as long as I could, never answering to my name when called, never acknowledging my existence. I would have gladly stayed in the dark. Weeks, months, years. And maybe I would've been forgotten. Maybe I would've become someone's good memory—"Remember that kid Ira? Best hider on the planet." Or, maybe, just maybe, the songs and stories about me would be absent of the word fat, would start first with *he loved the world too much, so he decided to vanish.*

"Open your eyes," Howard says.

The lights come on and the other students gather their things and there I lie, blinded by that sudden change, shocked back into the world, and for a second I forget about Body, forget its bulk, until I roll on my side and heave myself up.

8

🌸 🌸 🌸

Some days I take a shower in the dark. I keep the lights off, bring down the shades over the bathroom window, close the door. Taking a shower in the dark is not a conscious choice. I simply do it, and when the water hits me, when I grope for my shampoo and soap, I wonder why I decided on this act of cleaning myself without light. During these moments I realize Body sometimes makes his own decisions, moves on his own accord, imposes his own will. I read once that a man can see a fan spinning and he knows it will hurt but he can't stop his hand from touching the blades anyway. Experts say our bodies react to a set of neurological, psychological, and psychiatric conditions, that showering in the dark is a response to one or all of those conditions. Experts also say there is no difference between showering in the light and showering in the dark. But in the dark, I finally understand how well I know Body. My hand, without any visual cue, washes everything with care and precision, without pause. I slow down. I make sure every inch of Body—the dark crevices below the stomach and in between Body's legs—is covered with soap. In the light, the purpose of showering is to clean. In the dark, the purpose of showering is to explore.

🌸 🌸 🌸

We need reasons to explain who we are. We need reasons to explain our choices and decisions—good or bad.

But what if we don't have reasons? What if we stopped going to yoga because it made us too aware of ourselves, because it spotlighted our every flaw, because when we were asked to bend and contort, we couldn't? Instead of finding some sort of peace of mind, we found another activity Body had prevented us from enjoying.

So we stop.

We decide to do nothing. We decide to let Body take over. "Here you go, Body," we say. "Take the helm. Do your baddest." Body has been waiting for this moment. He has been clamoring for this opportunity, and now that he has it, he does nothing. Nothing is the best plan he can think of. Nothing is the fastest route to destruction.

Sometimes he speaks.

Sometimes Body says, "Downward-facing dog. Really?"

Sometimes Body says, "Remember that time you took yoga. What a joke."

So, we spend hours on the couch. We spend hours hating ourselves. We eat and eat and eat. We do this nonstop. We are killing ourselves but we can't stop. We hate ourselves but we don't say it. We want to die but we can't.

One, two, three. Four, five, six years speed by, and we are looking at the scale at the doctor's office. It reads three hundred ninety pounds. We are tired—so, so tired. This is the line we lean on. "How're you feeling?" the doctor says. "Tired," we say. "So, so tired." Could be the pounds we lug around. Could be the blood sugar we can't control. Could be the fact that most days are spent in one place.

We know what the doctor will say: lose weight, exercise. As a joke, we quote Raymond Carver's short story, "Fat": "Believe it or not, we have not always eaten this way." The doctor won't understand; most doctors don't. They are a breed who believe in logic and reason. To them, Body is about cause and effect. Body is about rational decisions. What he doesn't take into account is that our mind has become irrational. We ask for antidepressants. He looks at us and takes note. He asks if we are suicidal. We shake our head. He doesn't believe us. Why should he? Look at us. Look at the fat hanging over the chair. Look at our cheeks, our chins. He signs a prescription pad and then puts a hand on our shoulder. "Try this," he says. "Cut out a picture of a body you admire—a celebrity, perhaps, an athlete—and paste your face onto it. Hang it up so you look at it each day. Believe in the power of the mind."

We nod. We say this is a great idea. We thank him for his services.

Outside, the sun beats on us, and it is then we remember one yoga pose: Sun Salutation, a series of twelve moves consisting of lunging and bending and arching. We never got it right. But it didn't matter. Not that first time. Not any of the times. The point was we made Body move. We made Body realize it could be a flexible vessel, even when our sweat dripped onto the mat, even when our legs trembled, even when our stomach got in the way.

We're not saying this was the moment we would try again. We're not saying we went home and did not eat the mountain mound of rice. We ate. We're not saying we decided not to watch TV and opted for a walk instead. We watched. But something curious happened that day. We took the doctor's advice, but modified it. We took the body we envied—actor Brad Pitt—and cut out Brad's head and put it on our body. And now Brad Sukrungruang was doing the Sun Salutation. And now he was Downward Dogging. And now he was doing a headstand and realized what gravity does with fat. We laughed. Outside, in the summer heat, we laughed. Outside the doctor's office, we laughed. It sounded foreign from our mouth, but familiar, like the word *love* spoken in a different language.

❋ ❋ ❋

Body says, "Enough."

Body says, "My turn."

Body says, "I've got things to say, too."

Body says, "First, never again eat nacho cheese Combos." He reminds me of that day when we were in first grade and our mother bought Combos for the first time—such an ingenious concept, she thought, a tubular pretzel with cheese in the center—and we kept shoving our hands in the bag and popping them into our mouth.

Body says, "I gave you a warning after the fifteenth one."

Body says, "I learned a valuable lesson that day: you rarely listen." But those Combos, Body goes on, they were heavy in the stomach, so heavy the stomach wanted nothing to do with Combos, so up they came, up through the long and narrow esophagus and through the mouth and onto the green carpeted floor.

Body says, "Would it hurt to eat something green?"

Body knows that when I look in the mirror I see Body and cringe. When Body looks in the mirror, Body sees a boy who still doesn't understand limits, who insists on treating Body as if Body were expendable. Body knows that I am looking to point the finger. He understands it's easy to place blame, to put words in Body's mouth. Body wants to wrap his arm around me, push me into his flesh, two softnesses merging, melding. Body wants to whisper apologies.

Instead, Body says, "I am not to blame. I am only a body."

Body says, "It's time we stop talking."
Body says, "We need to make this work."
Body says, "It's time."

What prompted me to drive to the gym, I don't know. I woke one day in the fall, and instead of finding my spot on the couch, I got into the car, drove three miles east, and found myself in front of a gym. I didn't pause. I didn't hesitate as I had been doing for months, years, talking myself out of it, spinning and spinning my wheels. Perhaps it was the doctor and the diabetes and my wife and family. Perhaps it was vanity—pure vanity—because I would give anything to be skinny just once, to be lithe and bendable like Howard the yoga instructor. Perhaps it was my body that prompted change. Whatever it was, I was in a gym. I was taking aerobic classes. I was losing. Parts of me. Chunks of me. In a year, I lost over a hundred pounds. In a year, I found myself in the yoga studio again. There was a noticeable change in my body. Not just the weight and heft of it. Not just the space I occupied. This was a change that affected the air I took in.

Before she leads us into our first position, Maria, my new yoga instructor in Florida, tells the class to breathe deeply. She says we should prepare our bodies. My mat is in the front of the room. I sit, legs crossed, in baggy basketball shorts and a baseball cap. I take in air through my nostrils. My eyes are closed. I feel the air fill the inner cavity of my nose, feel it spread to every region of my body, down to the tip of my toes. I feel it enter my belly, a cool swirl like a tender wind. I remember once, back in the days when I lived in

13

upstate New York, back when Howard—bearded Howard—was my yoga instructor, I sat in the garden of my house, concentrating on my breath. Yoga breathing fascinated me. Like walking, I didn't realize there was a right way and a wrong way. But there I sat, eyes shut, breathing in and out. I took five breaths and opened my eyes. The world appeared brighter. Visually stunning. It was as if a gray film had been lifted from my eyes. I held on to this moment for as long I could. I kept breathing—oh, the joy of breathing!—and opening my eyes to a feast of color. The world moved, and I understood, only for this moment, that I was connected to it as Howard had been saying. I understood that you couldn't separate mind and body and spirit, that they acted in conjunction with one another. Then I realized I was becoming New Agey, and the thought made me self-conscious, and I was back to hating myself.

But I'm allowing for this. I'm allowing for vulnerability. I'm allowing for sadness. You can't stop it. You can only understand it.

Maria stands. I stand. She lifts her right foot. I lift mine. She places it against the other leg. So do I. And then we raise our arms straight into the air, lengthening our spines, opening our chests, our hearts, letting our fingers grow like branches. "Hold that pose," she says. "Feel how rooted you are to the earth." I do. I am a tree, for this moment, standing against a hard wind, knowing I will shake and tremble, but not fall.

Suzanne Morrison

Duet in Song and Smoke

It was the first day of 2013, and my mother and I were nearing the end of a New Year's walk around Green Lake, a pretty little puddle in the north end of the city that provides Seattleites with a perfect three-mile walk. We were preparing to move in the direction of a glass of wine when we both instinctively turned our heads toward the sound of some rather vigorous strumming. There, with the mirrored lake and wintering trees as his backdrop, a longhaired, bearded man wearing suspenders and a floppy, striped top hat serenaded the crowds soaking up the thin winter sun. He took breaks between chords to talk to the Rollerbladers, the mothers with strollers. As we passed, he said, quite blithely, as if just to my mother and me, "You know, everybody's always saying to me *It's All Good,* so I started saying it, too, *It's All Good,* I said, *It's All Good, Man,* but you know, it's not really true. I'm a Taoist so I know at least half of it's *All Bad.*"

We thought this was pretty funny. About a half mile earlier, my mother had told me she had breast cancer. All bad, indeed.

Over wine, my mother and I agreed that 2013 was off to a pretty lousy start. After she had told me everything she knew and I had absorbed the holy-fuck of it all, I went home, told my husband, called my siblings and my dad, and together we began the two-month-long process of waiting to know something, anything. Whether the prognosis would be good or bad, what type of cancer she had, how treatable it would be, whether it had spread anywhere, and finally, how we would fight it. How soon it would be done. This was what we talked about more than anything else: how quickly we could get this problem solved. My friend Erin laughed when I told her that: "That's the Morrison way," she said. "*Git 'er done!*"

In these days of pink ribbons and cancer walks, a breast cancer diagnosis is a curious thing. As my mother broke the news to her friends and coworkers, one after another said the same thing: Who *doesn't* have breast cancer? My mother was told that she was a future survivor, was given pink sports jerseys signed by local athletes, get-well cards full of ribbons. We comforted ourselves by reminding each other that our mother's got grit. That the doctors caught it early, and everyone knows if you catch it early, your chances of survival are extremely high. As cancers go, this was the one to get—the one with funding and screening and huge advancements in treatment.

I fully expected my mother to live for many years; this breast cancer, we agreed, would be a blip. The year 2013 would be a bad time we'd look back on and shake our heads. *That was tough,* we would say. No, I wasn't really scared that my mother would die. But I was terrified that she would change.

In theory, I love how suffering makes me stronger. I believe in learning from my injuries. In theory, I believe in suffering well, in turning my suffering over in my hands until I can see it from every angle, understand it, so that I may not be afraid of it. I know I have benefited from suffering when I've approached it with courage. In theory.

Real suffering, however? Real suffering can *suck it.* My own, but especially my mother's.

My mother, you see, is a force of nature. She was twenty when she and my father married, and for eight and a half years she didn't want children, wanted only to play the piano and enjoy a child-free adult life. But then, suddenly, she did want children, and within six years there were four of us scrabbling about on her floors. She was a talented musician, teaching and playing concerts all throughout my childhood. I grew up beneath her grand piano. I still get sleepy if I hear certain pieces by Tchaikovsky or Saint-Saëns, those she practiced at night after we had been put to bed.

When I was in high school, my parents hit a rough patch, financially, just as their four kids were launching, one by one, into college. So my mother channeled her musician's discipline into a master's in education, and then a principal's certificate. She became a vice principal at an elementary school, and then a principal, and eventually moved her way into administration until she was an associate superintendent of schools. She texts me messages after completing daylong hikes with my dad. She likes it when her hairdresser puts maroon highlights in her hair, says it makes her feel "kind of wild."

At sixty-six, she has a younger spirit than many of my friends. But the fear—oh my fear—was that she would emerge from a year of treatment changed, that my hale, vibrant mother would be reduced, aged, that surgeries and toxic drugs would make her slower. Older. More afraid.

Lurking beneath her brunette coif, my mother's actually got a full head of white hair. We joked that chemo would make it easy for her to transition from brunette to white; if she lost all her hair, she wouldn't have to do the embarrassing grow-out, wouldn't have to go to work with a head that looked tie-dyed. I laughed, but later that night, in bed, I fretted over the image of my mother white-headed and wizened after a year of treatment. I grieved the dark haired woman I've always known.

None of us slept well in January. By February, when an MRI revealed a second lump in her other breast, sleep became nearly impossible. When I did manage to drift off, it was into the lightest of dozes, and I dreamed of terrible things. Snakes and suffocation. Hissing vipers encircling my limbs like Laocoön's sea serpent, sinking their fangs into my arms and torso. In one dream, I covered my breasts, terrified that the vipers would bite me there. The largest snake squeezed my midsection until I couldn't breathe. Night after night, I awoke choking in the bedsheets, sucking in shallow, panicked gulps of cold air.

※ ※ ※

I'm still not entirely sure how I came to find myself in my first yoga class, back in late 2001, but I know I returned a few days later because I couldn't breathe. I was twenty-five and in a panic about pretty much everything—a looming move to New York, an insecure relationship, my grandparents' accelerating deterioration. The first time I remember losing my breath was when my grandfather was losing his; he had been a lifelong smoker and now, in his mid-eighties, had damaged his lungs and heart irreparably. Seeing my beloved, swearing-teddy-bear of a grandfather struggle for breath, I couldn't quite catch mine either.

In college, a drama professor had told me that smokers operated under the grave misconception that smoking relaxed us, when in fact it wasn't the cigarette at all but rather the deep, full breath one takes while pulling smoke into the lungs that gave one the smoker's calm. I remember being skeptical. I had started smoking at nineteen—old enough to know better—and had never been so calm. Finally, I had something to do with my hands. I had an excuse to leave a crowded party for ten minutes. I could sit by myself and not look alone. And I always had something to look forward to.

But by twenty-five, I couldn't help but notice how I smoked when I was stressed, in great big gulps of nicotine-laced air. The night my grandpa nearly stopped breathing on me, I went home and smoked a half pack of cigarettes. The next day I went to yoga and gratefully breathed through round after round of bhastrika, imagining myself cleansing the smoke and tar from my lungs, wishing I could send those big round breaths to my grandfather's lungs.

For most of my adult life, yoga and smoking were my yin and my yang. I was always doing one or the other: if I was in a healthy state of mind, I did yoga. The second life turned on me, I smoked. Maybe that sounds self-destructive, and maybe it was, but in my truest heart,

I think smoking was a survival technique. All through the tumult of my twenties, I needed something to look forward to, and every hour or so, there was a cigarette. During bad times, I lived from one cigarette to the next, obsessively writing in journals, until I knew every aspect of what was wrong, until I had studied my loss or fear so thoroughly I could finally set it aside. And of course, smoking felt glamorous, and nothing makes suffering as bearable as a little glamour. Would yoga have been better? Sure. Probably. But I always knew I was getting better when I wanted to stretch. When my craving switched from cigarettes to pranayama.

Waiting for one test result after another this winter, 2013, the winter my mother was diagnosed, was the first time in my adult life I didn't turn to cigarettes in my time of need. I practiced yoga, and those ninety-minute packages of breathing and asana, they helped. But, honestly? Not enough. If only I could have smoked! The crazy thing was, I didn't want to. Writing this is the first time it's even occurred to me that in earlier years I would've depleted box after box of Camels.

I quit for good three years ago. The only time I've smoked in all that time was for a promotional trailer for my book, *Yoga Bitch*, and even then, it was just for show. I didn't even inhale. (This fact made one of my smoking friends look at me as if she had just learned I was a Cylon.)

My grandmother once told me that she quit smoking on a whim, that, at sixty, she put out a cigarette after dinner one night and simply decided she didn't want to smoke anymore. So I wasn't too surprised when three years ago it occurred to me—simply *occurred* to me, this was neither a decision nor an epiphany—that I didn't want to smoke anymore. And I haven't, not once, in the three years since then. I've done a lot of yoga, and when I've been sad, or scared, I have sat with it, unglamorously miserable, reminding myself to breathe.

In the fall of 2004, at twenty-eight, I quit the only corporate job I had ever held in order to write, and promptly came down with a phantom lung condition. This was a job that had been meant to get me set up in New York, which I took to pay off debt, get an apartment, and save up enough money to be able to quit and write full time for a while. I even marked my calendar for six months and one year from my start date, with the letters: QJ? Which stood for "Quit Job?"

Most of my friends and family made fun of me for my rather constant preoccupation with quitting the best job I'd had in my life. By best job, I mean that it paid me 47K a year, provided me with medical, dental, and vision insurance, and I didn't have to do anything except send excremental instant messages to my friends for eight hours a day. By excremental IMs, I mean that there were days when there was so little to do and so much had already been gossiped about over IM that a few friends and I would resort to writing the word *POOP* in different fonts and colors, sending these messages back and forth for hours at a time.

It was the easiest job ever to pay me so well. Every other job I had known had, at one time or another, required me to actually *work*. But this job's biggest requirement was rhetoric. Memorizing Core Values like *entrepreneurship* and *diversity,* both of which had personal and professional equivalents that we were supposed to embody, one beige day after another.

Everyone told me I was crazy when I quit. Everybody told me that you wait to sell a book first, *then* you quit your day job. And if any of them had read the manuscript I had saved on my laptop at that point, they would have been all the more adamant: *do not DO NOT quit your day job.*

I quit in a sort of backhanded way; I tend to slither out of doors before slamming them shut behind me. I first took a short-term leave of absence in order to go home to Seattle and work on the book there, after which I could return to work or quit for good. While I was home in Seattle, my grandfather's lungs finally gave out on him, and rather than write, I spent my days with my siblings and friends, smoking cigarettes, drinking coffee, talking about grandpa, dreaming about the day I could move home. When I returned to New York, I took a leap of faith and told HR I wouldn't be returning to my desk. I forfeited my salary and health insurance. I vowed to stay unemployed until I had a finished book.

Every day, I sat in my room with my laptop, working. The super dropped off a notice warning us that the management company had laced our walls with poison; that the sweetish smell seeping from the walls came from decomposing rodents; that it would be gone when they were. I lit candles to mask the smell and wrote like a motherfucker, taking breaks to check in on the 2004 election. In the evening, when my boyfriend came home from work, I followed him around the apartment like an annoying dog, hungry for conversation after a day of solitude, while he longed for peace and quiet after a day out in the world.

I hadn't spent so much time alone in years. It was exactly what I wanted, but it was changing me. When I looked up from my computer screen after hours of work, my life looked strange. For the first time, I was doing something I had always wanted to do. What else did I want? What else, I wondered, could I do?

By the time Bush was reelected, I had completed a draft of my novel. I had a relationship with an interested agent. And I couldn't breathe.

Naturally, I figured it was cancer. I was going through a nonsmoking phase, but even so. My brother Frank sent me one of his inhalers. "It's not cancer," he said. "You've probably got asthma."

My friend Jean-Michele hooked me up with a Russian doctor she had heard about, a friend of a friend who gave breaks to artists and was a little bit famous for giving enormous shots of penicillin and vitamin B for anything that might ail you. In her cramped, dingy exam room, a three-sided cubicle with a ripped shower curtain for a door, I studied the clippings and photographs tacked up to the walls while her one-eyed assistant (no joke) stabbed at my vein with a butterfly syringe till she drew blood, then hooked me up to the tentacles of an EKG machine and left me alone.

Every inch of the cubicle walls fluttered with clippings from medical journals, business cards of legal reps, and dozens of small prints of Russian paintings. I counted three articles bearing titles such as "Medical research finds that drinking improves cognitive function of women" and "Two drinks a day may keep the neurologist away."

Two photographs caught my eye, both of a woman in a pink unitard exhibiting yoga poses on a pink yoga mat. Headstand and Bridge. The photographs were taped to a piece of pink construction paper. I was a bit of an Iyengar fascist at the time, convinced there was a right and a wrong way to do every pose, and I instantly set about critiquing the woman's alignment in the postures. She looked a little bit stiff. My yogic mantras, then and always, were: *Strong but soft. Difficult yet easy.* Judgey, judgey. I noticed some words between the two pictures. They were written in a thin black pen, and the handwriting was close to illegible. But I could make out "Mrs. Conrad, 95 years old."

Finally the doctor arrived, a large woman with frizzy auburn hair and a gauze bandage wrapped many times around her neck. I tried not to look at the bandage as I told her that I felt like I was wearing a corset. That I woke up at night feeling strangled. That I could never quite catch my breath. After reviewing my EKG, she told me, in her thick, sticky Russian accent, that there was nothing wrong with me but unhappiness.

"No one loves you in New York," she said. "Your boyfriend, maybe, but your family, your brother with the asthma, they are not here, and they are the ones who love you. And so you panic. Here, New Yorkers, they smile at you with their faces but they do not care about you."

She prescribed two things for my inability to breathe: Xanax, and daily, hour-long walks. And just before she drew the shower curtain away from the wall to leave, she mentioned that I might consider singing, if it was the sort of thing I did. "Singing helps you breathe," she said.

I didn't fill the prescription, I took exactly one walk, and I never sang. But six months later I left my boyfriend, my brand-new law firm job, and New York, and returned to my family. To my brother with the asthma. I returned to Seattle, where I knew I was loved. And after a while, it seemed I could breathe again.

☙ ☙ ☙

At the beginning of 2012, we lost a dear family friend, the man who was my sister's godfather, who had been like an uncle or a surrogate father to me. He and his wife were my parents' best friends, their children were like three extra siblings. George had been diagnosed with liver cancer shortly before I moved home from New York. Still, he lived for seven years, through surgeries and chemo; he knew three of his granddaughters, and died a few weeks after meeting his fourth, his namesake, Georgia. Not long after we got the news, his daughter Emily told my sister and me that George had wanted us to sing at his memorial service. She and her siblings wanted comforting, uplifting songs, nothing too sad. Of course we said we would do it, but we were both more than a little nervous.

When asked if we still sing, my sister and I have often joked that we do weddings and funerals, otherwise, never. We both took voice lessons for years, sang in choirs from elementary school on. We have both sung on the stage of the Seattle Opera. My sister even considered making opera her career, and she probably could have: her voice is both better and bigger than mine. But her stint at Seattle Opera convinced her to go into journalism instead. Most singers, she said at the time, shuddering, are as narcissistic as actors, but *Christian*. Actors, she could take. Christians too. But the combination, she said, was impossible; she'd rather cover Congress. For my part, I enjoyed occasional fantasies about becoming a professional singer, but I also knew that music wasn't my calling; I had too modest a talent and none of the discipline for it. But Jill and I have always sung together, and usually at weddings and funerals. I sing soprano, Jill mezzo. Our voices are very similar, though Jill's shades dark, mine light.

All through our twenties, we crashed our performances. I was in New York and Jill was in Seattle, or Jill was in Washington, DC, and I was in Seattle, and we would decide by email or phone which duets in our repertoire we would sing at which function, and then, usually the night before or the morning of the wedding or funeral, we would sing smoky scales, arpeggios ripping through the cobwebs in our lungs until a clear tone emerged, at which point we knew we were ready to go. Somehow we always managed to pull it off, though I sweated through my highest notes and neither of us had enough control over our breath to achieve the more subtle effects that would make a piece of music really soar. Still, we managed. We had been trained well. Our mother always accompanied us on the piano, and afterward she would remind us of how good we could be, if we just applied ourselves again. If we stopped smoking.

The songs we sang in those days were classical or musical theater standards we could do in our sleep: "Panis Angelicus," "Pie Jesu"; we sang the simple "Edelweiss" in two-part harmony at my grandmother's funeral, because she had loved it. The three of us—my mother, my sister, and I—had done this so many times.

Somehow, a couple of years had passed without a wedding or a funeral performance. Now, for George, we wanted to do our best, but we were as out of shape as we'd ever been. Sure, we'd both quit smoking, but that didn't mean either of us had begun singing daily scales. What we were most sure of was that we needed to be confident in our songs, because this was a different sort of funeral; so far, we had sung at the funerals of elderly grandparents. This time, we would watch our oldest friends grieve. Our parents had lost a dear friend. In losing George we had the first taste of what it would be like to lose our own father or mother. We were going to have to be strong to get through the performance without breaking down.

We chose the "Panis Angelicus" for our second piece, because we could do it in our sleep. But for the opening song, the one we would sing as the family lit candles on the altar, we chose the "Evening Prayer" from Humperdinck's *Hansel and Gretel*. My sister had sung the part of Hansel years earlier, when she worked for the Seattle Opera. In high school, I had sung in the chorus, and had sat every night, rapt, as two honest-to-god opera stars sang that gorgeous duet, their voices braiding together in the hushed opera house like silver and gold ropes. The duet arrives at the end of Act II, as Hansel and Gretel make a bed for themselves in the dark forest, and pray to the angels to keep them safe:

> *When at night I go to sleep*
> *Fourteen angels watch do keep*
> *Two my head are guarding*
> *Two my feet are guiding . . .*

The first time my mother and I ran through my part, a month before the memorial service, I couldn't hit the high notes and I couldn't make it through a full verse without crying. If you've ever tried to sing and cry at the same time, you'll know how well that works. The tones come out strangled, you make all kinds of squeaking, snuffling, mortifying sounds. If I was going to get through this song without breaking down, I would have to be both strong and open: strong enough physically to support those high notes with my fullest breath, and strong enough emotionally to keep my throat open and soft. That was the only way to give the music the kind of expression it deserved, to make the notes and words beautiful. Strength in softness, softening in strength: I knew this challenge well. I had been doing it for over a decade in yoga.

I made it to yoga class maybe once a week that winter, but when I did, I focused all my attention on my diaphragm. I had grown lazy in my practice, allowing my mind to wander in poses that had long ago become easy. Now I focused on that rubber band just below my rib cage. I stretched from the triangular hollow at my center, the entrance to my diaphragm's cave. I needed that part of my body more than I ever had. It was what would get me through George's funeral without breaking down. It was what would help me ascend those scales. The more I focused on my breathing, the calmer I felt. Each day I found ten minutes, twenty minutes, sometimes more, to sing the scales I hadn't sung in years. I summoned every lesson my voice teachers had ever given me. I smiled when I sang; it makes the tone prettier. I imagined my rib cage as a cathedral full of space, my voice bouncing off the acoustical architecture just behind my cheekbones. Every day my voice was stronger, clearer, and I felt stronger and clearer as well. I went to yoga more often. I remembered how freeing discipline can be.

The day of the memorial came, and my sister and I stood on the altar of the Presbyterian church George had attended for decades. We stood in front of the people gathered to mourn, and we sang. We watched our friends walk together, hand in hand, down the center aisle of the church, watched them light candles around George's picture. We looked to each other for strength, to keep our voices blending. We listened for our mother's piano just beneath our voices, and we breathed. I felt my eyes tear up, but my throat stayed open, and the notes poured forth. I listened to my sister, to my mother, and they listened to me. Together, we sang a song of comfort. A song of angels.

✿ ✿ ✿

Throughout this winter, as my mother's doctors debated lumpectomy vs. mastectomy, radiation vs. hormone therapy vs. chemo; as I rejected, again and again, the thought of my mother's mortality, the image of a surgeon cutting into my mother's body, cutting open that part of her I once claimed as my own; throughout all of that, I had terrible dreams. But once, I dreamed of George. His death had just hit the one-year mark.

It started as one of the same dreams I'd suffered all winter. Snakes, suffocation. I could smell things in these dreams. Rotting rodents. Dust. The soap on a surgeon's hands. This time, I was in a hospital and the doctor told me that my sister and I had breast cancer, but that mine was "regressive," which, in my dream world, meant it had spread through my entire body. I wouldn't last the night. Soon people started showing up to say goodbye to me, and my husband, Kurt, was crying, and I was thinking: well, at least I can die while Kurt holds me. That will be a nice way to go out. And then I left the room, and George was in the hallway, dapper in a tuxedo shirt and pants, and he told me he didn't want to stay long or see anybody else, but that everything was going to be OK. Then he held me and I sobbed until I couldn't breathe.

I woke up, as I had done so many times that week, gasping. It was already midmorning, nearly noon, and my husband was gone for the day. I had the house to myself. I felt foggy, thick, exhausted. Checked my phone for texts from my mom or dad, looked at my email for the same, and, finding nothing, turned them both off. We were waiting for the results of an MRI that would tell us if the second lump was cancerous. I started to make tea.

Sometimes, while my tea is brewing, I wander over to my grandmother's piano, which I inherited, and play a bit of a prelude or sonata. Whenever I've been sad, I tend to play the piano. I know some very sad songs. When I left New York, I played Chopin's Prelude No. 4, the one that was played at his funeral, every day for a year. But today my fingers were cold. And I wasn't sad; I was scared.

There is a photograph of George on my piano, looking handsome in a tux, standing next to my sister on her wedding day. I thought of the gift he gave me by requesting that we sing at his funeral. That request had brought something beautiful back into my life. I felt the paralysis in my diaphragm, the seizure there that was so familiar, that made my breathing shallow and forced, that kept my breath from cresting the way I needed it to in order to relax. George had given me a way to breathe again. I touched my finger to Middle C, and sang a scale. Then C-sharp, another scale. D, D-sharp, E. My mother taught me those notes before I knew the alphabet. Now, I filled my house with them, with her, with song.

Adriana Páramo

Sitting Doggietation and the Unknown Knowns

I am in Somerset, England, ten minutes away from Bath and a short drive west of Stonehenge. I stand, alone and out of place, in the vestibule of a stately 300-year-old Victorian mansion built on 550 acres of parklands and lakes, a space with history and an Elizabethan air: boudoirs and stone fireplaces. I am wearing an expensive dress, black nylons, and high heels. My hair is up in a loose ponytail tied with a bow made out of braids, with whimsical curls the same color as my hair. Little crystal chandeliers dangle from my ears, giving out rays of light like ocean beacons. I look the part.

The wedding organizer escorts the parents of the bride out of the cocktail room and toward the spiral staircase for the photo session.

The door is left ajar. I see them. Leah holds hands with her husband. They have been married for ten minutes. Behind them stand her parents: my husband and his ex-wife. They would have been married thirty-three years. The four of them look straight into the camera and smile with joy. I feel my chest heave. *Samma vayama*, I repeat in my head. I invoke the sixth Buddhist path, the one about Right Effort, the one that teaches that in order to avoid suffering, I must promote good thinking and conquer evil thoughts. The photographer snaps more pictures and asks Leah's brother to join in; now the family is complete for the picture. Their lives pass before my eyes in snapshots of a past that doesn't belong to me. It's theirs, it is history written with Play-Doh and scraped knees, with tickles and tears, with first loves and diaries, with birthday cakes, anniversaries, vacations, report cards, graduations, family life. It's history written on Mary's body: the healthy one she once had, with evenings of shaved legs, perfume behind her ears, and orgasms, and the one weakened by cancer she inhabits now, with chemotherapy rounds, thinning veins, and a bald head. I close the door and grab a glass of champagne that I don't drink but gives me something to occupy my hands. I walk around wishing to disappear, to be the unknown guest, to melt into the fluid continuum of the grandiose drapery around me and not to be noticed. But here, everyone seems to know who I am.

The woman who split the bride's parents apart.

The man-eating Latina who seduced Mary's husband.

Someone talks to me in a thick English accent that I don't understand. I ignore him or her and keep walking. I get a few dirty looks. My shoulders rise and fall, rise and fall, in choppy outbursts of contained sobs. *Samma vayama. Samma vayama,* I whisper under my breath as I hear my husband's laughter coming from the staircase outside. I wonder what's making him laugh. Is Mary laughing with him? Did they just remember a private joke? Why is he laughing? Why? What kind of secret code do couples forge after decades of being together? Why did I ever think it was possible to ignore the massive weight of my husband's past? To disregard what Slovenian philosopher Slavoj Žižek called "the unknown knowns," the things that we know but have forgotten, the things that we know but are unaware of knowing?

My mouth feels dry and my tongue is pasty. I need Thich Nhat Hanh's words, I need a rosary, a mala, a pebble. I need my dog.

⚜ ⚜ ⚜

To say that I'm a Buddhist would be a stretch. I don't believe in reincarnation, I interpret Buddhism's five precepts as mere guidelines, I have nonvirtuous thoughts, lots of them, I gossip, lie, and have no moral qualms about squashing a bloodsucking mosquito smack on any part of my body. Yet, ever since I took my first Buddhism 101 class back in the early 90s, since Thich Nhat Hanh, the Vietnamese monk, spoke to me through his books, since I found out that being good is the biggest challenge I will ever face, I've been calling myself a Buddhist. And then of course there is the business of samadhi, concentration, meditation, and a quiet mind, which if observed, preferably sitting padmasana-style—in full lotus—is supposed to lead me to personal freedom. A stern yoga practitioner I once met, concerned with my lax interpretation of Buddhism, wrote down, in Sanskrit of course, the sequence of asanas for me to follow in order to conquer the coveted padmasana: Virabhadrasana II, followed by Utthita Parsvakonasana, followed by Utthita Trikonasana. Or a combination of Janu Sirsasana and Ardha Matsyandrasana Marichyasana. I laughed when she gave me the paper, thinking that she was joking. She was dead serious.

Over the years, many friends have come to my aid with ideas on how to meditate effectively so that my monkey mind actually quiets. Focus on a triangle, visualize light, eliminate the terrestrial, strive for the outwardly. Or the opposite: welcome every noise you hear, put your senses on high alert. Breathe, hold, exhale. Straighten your spine, open each of your seven chakras, activate your kundalini. To no avail. I don't have a monkey mind. What I have in my brain is a whole zoo of locked-up creatures strung out on Ecstasy: any attempt at quieting them only seems to unlock their cages, to let them run wild and free up and down the corners of my cerebral cortex. But that's a thing of the past. I got rid of the full lotus and the chakras and the triangle, forgot about the kundalini and gave up on counting my breaths. Now I tame the little creatures with sitting doggietation.

I start small and unassuming. Usually with a sigh. Hers, not mine. Honey has a broad face and neck like a pit bull and light caramel fur like a yellow Labrador. She lies on a blanket over her bed and rearranges herself until she is completely comfortable, which in her case means what I call Super Honey to the Rescue Position, stretched out the length of her bed, on her stomach, looking like she is either flying or ready to go as soon as she hears me move. I sit in my comfy chair and remain as immobile as possible, trying not to wink. Then we have a stare down. We examine each other silently. The slightest movement on my part can be interpreted as a call to action, make her wag her tail, or change position, or scratch her face, or lick her backside. I stare attentively, not thinking, not trying not to think; go deep into her eyes, the color of freshly minted pennies, until her eyelids get heavy and her eyes start to close with boredom and disinterest. She dozes off, blinks weightily, once, twice, then falls asleep. I start to meditate. I focus my attention on her right ear, that floppy origami of cartilage and hair that folds above her right eye. I imagine what a furry ear above my own right eye must feel like. I welcome the soft moss of warm fur on my forehead. Honey exhales. I exhale after her. She takes a long deep breath, holds it, then lets go noisily through her mouth. Her jowls reverberate quietly. I let out a *ptfff.* An ambulance zooms by; the shrill of the siren is a distant echo under my floppy ear. She rests her head on one of her paws. I know exactly the kind of smell she is inhaling. Throughout the years I have made her paws my acquaintances. I have washed them, I have cured sores and removed ticks, I have tickled them, caressed them, massaged them. Honey's paws smell of the Saint Augustine grass in our backyard, of bread crumbs left on our kitchen floor, of the wine one of us spilled the night before. Her paws smell of home, of this life I have built with my husband.

The last time I saw Mary, I was having an affair with her husband. She found us having coffee at my place. It wasn't a love triangle by any measure. It was more like a heptagon. I was married and had a child in sixth grade, they had two children in boarding school. It was a complicated mess. I was on a four-year teaching contract; he was on a four-year assignment with the British Army. Oh, and we lived in a Muslim country. Mary vowed to destroy me, to divulge our dirty little secret to his brigadier, to my school principal, to everyone in Kuwait. No corners of my man-eating life would be untouched by her wrath. She spat her venom upon me as I held the door open for her, as we walked down the hallway. I will destroy you, she swore, walking into my kitchen, ready to confront her husband, my lover. I understood at that moment that I had lost control over my life and that Mary had the power to cause as much or as little pain as she deemed necessary. After that encounter I lived every day afraid she'd expose me, make me lose my job, my crumbling marriage, the order I was trying so hard to maintain. She fought to defend what was hers: her family, her husband, certainty, comfort, a future. She fought as any woman would: with her heart and her mouth, with fire and rage and love. And when she finally understood that there was nothing that her mouth or her heart could do to mend her marriage, she left the country, taking my secret, our secret, with her.

Honey is a mutt, a hodgepodge of breeds, rescued from the pound twelve years ago when she was a puppy. We knew she was the one the moment we saw her. She licked my daughter's face through the bars of the cage, wagged her tail when my husband knelt next to my daughter. I stood behind them and for a fleeting moment I believed we were a family getting a puppy rather than remnants of two previous families trying hard and clumsily to build our own. We got Honey and my daughter remained my daughter and my husband remained my husband, but we were never a family.

I haven't seen or spoken to Mary in fifteen years, since the day in my kitchen. Today, as the guests move in and out of the mansion, we end up facing each other by the house entrance overlooking a lake. I reach out to hold her hands, the way older women do, fully expecting her to leave me there with hands wide open. She holds my hands in return and we exchange pleasantries. I congratulate her on Leah's marriage, tell her she looks great, compliment her outfit and the venue. She smiles, and her cheeks look impossibly high for a woman touching fifty. I look for anger in her eyes. I find none. I suspect she has been simmering this little act for fifteen years: be nice, smile, wait for it, wait for it, then blow up when more guests gather around, give the homewrecker a piece of your mind when the audience grows. A plan I perfectly understand. If I were her, I'd wait for the right moment too; I would humiliate me publicly and stridently like a glass castle imploding on itself.

After the photo session, the wedding coordinator beckons everyone to the dining room. Everything is perfect. The centerpieces, the food, the smiley guests, the tables, all of them round except the one reserved for the couple. The couples. At the rectangular table sit the newlyweds and their parents. My husband has just delivered his father-of-the-bride speech and beams with joy as he replenishes four champagne flutes, one for Leah, one for the groom, one for himself, and one for his ex-wife. Did he touch her arm as he offered her more champagne? Is her skin as smooth as it looks? Did he feel her skin and think, Oh, I remember this, how lovely. And when she looked up to say, Yes, please, that'd be nice, could he smell her breath? Did he notice how white her teeth are and how demure her smile is? Did he hear her London accent and think, Oh, how much I miss her Queen's English?

Something is welling up in me, a dust devil is whirling faster and faster, growing bigger and bigger. I think I just let out a whimper. Are you okay? someone at the table asks me. Yes, of course. Weddings make me emotional, I say as I wipe the corners of my eyes with the tip of my napkin. I excuse myself. I need to regroup. To remember my place. To purify and calm my mind so that I can muster a sliver of *prajna*, discernment, insight, wisdom. I remember Thich Nhat Hanh's words in his book about anger: "The Buddha never advised us to suppress our anger. He taught us to go back to ourselves and take good care of it." I need to take care of this wind before it becomes a tornado.

On my way out of the wedding hall I look over at the main table. My husband is dressed in tails; his ex-wife is wearing a purple ensemble complemented with a feathery fascinator, a lacy bit hangs over one side of her forehead. She looks gorgeous.

I walk along a wall-to-wall antique mirror adorning the hall outside the dining room. By the time I start climbing the spiral staircase leading to our bedroom overlooking the estate's eighteen-hole golf course, tears are streaming down my face, rivulets of black mascara forming a gravity-defying lagoon at the tip of my chin. I dredge every residual chunk of self-esteem from the Mariana depths of my raging-with-jealousy heart. I climb the stairs faster.

Honey was spayed at the SPCA before we adopted her. My husband had a vasectomy when he was married to Mary. How odd, I think, that these two beings I adore are sterile. My husband and I will have neither puppies nor babies. But this acknowledgement of the end of our reproductive lives doesn't keep me from imagining little bronzed things with blue eyes running around the house. Our children. How I love the sound and the idea of those two words together: Our. Children. His and Mine. I read somewhere that sometimes spayed dogs experience phantom heats. Some residual primal instinct kicks in, setting their barren wombs ablaze, and the poor things walk around sniffing, looking for a male to mate with, bearing the full weight of the kind of loneliness that only a human could understand. No man has ever deserted me, but I understand the longing, that sticky sadness of a bed too big for one, the unbearable stillness of lonely mornings filled with nothing but cold coffee, the accusatory silence of a telephone that doesn't ring, the wrinkles that, one day, turn up around the eyes like unwanted guests, the recognition that one's marriage is over and that the father of your children is in the arms of another woman.

I also read that domesticated dogs are highly promiscuous. When in heat, they readily mate with multiple partners, and since humans provide the necessities to grant the survival of the litter, a dog no longer needs to form a social bond with its mate. I can't resist the temptation to give Honey human attributes. Because of me, I reflect, she will never be a mother, she will never have a partner, a family. Because of the decisions I made, the four of us—my husband, Mary, my ex-husband, and me—all in our forties and fifties now, will die without a nuclear family.

My dog, my companion, is getting old. Her golden stop and muzzle used to remind me of fields of wheat, sugar cane syrups and marigolds. Now they are gray, a constant reminder of my own aging process. I am getting old. Together we age, and together we meditate. I visualize her 320 bones expanding and contracting with each breath she takes. I think of my 206 parts moving in and out of themselves as I breathe. She lies on her back, exposing the scar on her belly. I have a similar scar on mine, courtesy of an invasive endometriosis case. My body sinks into the chair, then spreads out like a puddle of oil. Nothing exists but a middle-aged woman with one ovary and a barren dog. The lake outside our home loses its water and with it, its flora and its sentient inhabitants. The tropical verdure of our garden slowly dissipates in a vacuum of dog's inhalations and a light snore. Honey's eyes move rapidly under her three sets of eyelids. I cradle my eyes in their sockets and turn them down to gaze at Honey's whiskers as I reflect on the Buddha's Four Noble Truths on human suffering.

Dukkha: *Suffering exists.* Last year, when Leah called my husband to tell him that Mary was dying of cancer, I took Honey to my writing room and wept. I knew it wasn't my fault, but somehow I felt responsible. It should have been me, the one fighting for her life; I, who destroyed their family, should be the one punished with cell-killing matter, my body bombarded with death squadrons gnawing at my colon, not hers. If what Buddhism teaches about karmic law is true, I thought, I should be the one getting radiated, my curls falling out in chunks, my skin getting blotched with phantom cinders of molecular ions. I, the ex-smoker, ex-drinker, ex-pothead, ex-Catholic. I, the cheating wife, the lousy mother, the detached daughter, the pottymouth. Not Mary. Leah and the groom decided to bring the wedding forward and get married six months earlier than initially planned. The invitation is for both of us, my husband said. You're coming with me, right? Of course not, I said.

Samudaya: *There is a cause for suffering.* I had an irrational desire to control the situation. I imagined healing Mary one meditation session at a time, exorcising the pain, casting the malignant cells off her body with the sheer power of my mindful doggietation. I caressed Honey's hackles with determination, with faith, with anguish. I wanted to infuse life into her and therefore into Mary's ailing body. I turned Honey on her back and massaged her belly, that jiggly mass of teats, scars, and summer rashes, whispering spontaneous healing prayers into her mossy ears. Get well, please, get well. I talked to her cancer: Go away, leave her alone, she doesn't deserve you. I combed Honey's withers with my fingers, feeling a type of devotion I didn't know I had in me. Don't die, please, don't die.

Nirodha: *There is an end to suffering.* The mind lets go of any desire or craving. Three months before the wedding, I dreamed about Mary. We were at a little street café in Paris. We weren't talking; we seemed to know each other's words before they were uttered, because by virtue of giving our love to the same man, we had become soul sisters. She had lost her hair and this made her feel naked and ashamed. Without words, somehow, I told her that I'd shave my head in solidarity if that meant anything to her. She smiled. I reached over to caress her bald head, but just as I was about to touch her, I woke up. And I felt lighter and filled with renewed fortitude. I interpreted this dream as an omen. It dispelled any doubts about whether or not I should attend Leah's wedding. I was ready to go. Mary was dying. Mary had lost her hair during her second round of chemotherapy. Her cancer had spread to organs beyond the colon. I was alive, younger, with a head bursting with curls. I was fit and healthy. If she wanted to slap me in public and spit whatever residual venom she might still have after fifteen years, I could take it. I was stronger than she was.

Magga: *In order to end suffering, you must follow the Eightfold Path.* I trained my heart for the wedding the way an athlete trains for a triathlon. I worked on my *samma ditthi*, or Right View. I figured that if I could see through Mary's anger, if I could grasp the impermanent and imperfect nature of love and understand the law of karmic conditioning, I would attain understanding of the true nature of all things. She'll be angry, I'll be compassionate. She'll want revenge, I'll offer her understanding. She'll blame me for everything that had gone wrong in her life, I'll accept responsibility.

Once I decided to attend Leah's wedding, I incorporated into my doggietation sessions a relentless journey toward *samma sankappa*, Right Intention, the volitional aspect of my mind that controls my actions. I committed myself to ethical and mental self-improvement. I would resist the pull of desire, anger, and aversion. I would not think or act cruelly, violently, or aggressively. I would develop compassion. I was determined to be the best human being I could possibly be.

I trained deliriously. My mind and heart slowly melted into a peaceful continuum. I fervently focused my attention on Honey's breath, therefore on mine, and used it as the means of spreading kindness and goodwill. I visualized our breaths as one ray of light gradually sweeping over my body. I directed patient kindness toward myself, with the thought *If I open my heart, Mary will open hers*, and let the mood of that thought spread outward from the heart, through the body, through the mind and beyond myself.

I was ready. I started packing for England.

Alone in our room I burst into sobs. I am my husband's wife. I didn't take his last name when we got married because I didn't want to become anything other than the woman my mother named after a beauty queen in the 60s, but I'm his wife. The wife. And right at this moment that's all I want people to acknowledge. It's a childish thought, a shallow need to have my ego stroked. I know this. But before I know it, I start making a mental list of who I'm not. I'm not British, I'm not Mrs. Macklin, I'm not the mother of those two well-adjusted young adults, I'm not their stepmother either. I'm an indelible blemish on their family history, a wife who can exist only on the periphery of their lives. A long list of unknown knowns.

I kick off my shoes, remove my nylons and the bow in my hair. I lie flat on the cold wooden floor and play dead, my futile attempt at impromptu Savasana, the only yoga posture I have the energy for. I align my body, make sure that both sides rest evenly on the floor. The wood creaks under my weight. I think of Honey, my vehicle to blissful neutrality. I conjure up her Super Honey to the Rescue Pose and let the boundaries of my own body dissolve and melt into her ashy stop. I take refuge in her grey hackles, exhale noisily, stop crying, work on calming my senses. I strive for *samma sati,* Right Mindfulness, and the moment I become aware of my body, my mind and my feelings, I begin to cry again, this time more violently than before.

Finally, I surrender any and all psychological effort. I drop my brain to the back of the skull and see me for who I am rather than for who I wanted to be. I came to this party puffed up with rhetorical mindfulness. I trained my body and mind, striving for moral superiority—not to attain, maintain, or spread compassion. I accepted the invitation to attend Leah's wedding so that I could put my boundless kindness on display, so that I could rub my highly sophisticated spirit in the faces of anyone looking my way, anyone judging me. But more than anything, I had envisioned my meeting with Mary as a battlefield, a chess game where I'd be the willing martyr. I'd sacrifice my pride for her benefit, I'd offer her the other cheek after she strikes square and bold across the face, and everyone would look at me and say, She is one hell of a woman, so spiritually advanced.

Buddhism and yoga teach that the best place is right here, this moment. I let the tears form puddles in the crevasses of my ears. I remember the Zen practice called shikantaza, Just Sit Hit Mind, the constant return to the direct experience of whatever is "hitting mind." What's hitting mine is the party going on downstairs, the physical source of my immediate suffering. I use an image of Honey to redirect my mind. Sometimes when I doggietate, she lies on her back and her flews hang lifelessly at the corners of her mouth, exposing a pink gum sprinkled with spots that are brown, asymmetrical, and capriciously distributed, a fact that doesn't cease to amaze me because it reminds me of her true nature, it represents what she is: a mutt, all the dog breeds and none. In that position, her teeth are fully exposed. Honey has what's known as a bulldog bite, an underbite: six jagged lower incisors covering their upper jaw counterparts. Framing her two sets of incisors are her canines. They are wolf-looking fangs, long, thick, powerful. Highly specialized structures which serve as weapons of offense and defense, sharp cuspids designed to grab, cut, and crush. Yet I put my hand between her jaws, I place my forearm across her open mouth, testing her, challenging her inner wild wolf to come out. She is never interested. She pulls gently away from me as if saying, There you go again, you and your lame tests; how many times do I have to tell you I will never hurt you? This thought makes my mind wander off again. Not downstairs, but to that day, fifteen years ago, when Mary left Kuwait, quietly, in complete and utter surrender.

And just like that, the quintessential unknown known punches me nice and square in my throat. I'm more flawed than I ever thought possible. Oh, dear God, I'm disgusting, I say to no one as I sit in half lotus. I expected to see a dying woman, frail and bald, her skin discolored and withered by radiation, her eyes sunken with pain, her lips chapped and blistered at the corners, her hands mangled with needle marks and worry. She was none of this. She looked amazingly radiant and she was neither angry nor revengeful. She is a better woman than me; she has become, without my Buddhist sophistry, the best human being she can be. The only one who's been haunted by the past is me. The only one clinging to delusion has been the one training feverishly to avoid it. Me. I thought Mary had carried the heavy cross of anger for fifteen years, but it was me who carried it for her, not of anger but guilt. I bring my legs against my chest, rest my chin on my knees, and cry in shame.

I don't know this yet, but in a few minutes my husband will come looking for me. He'll find me disheveled, with mascara smudged down my face, my lips colorless and my hair limp with sweat and tears. The sight will confuse him. He won't understand anything because I won't tell him what I just found out about myself. I won't tell him that I'm not as good a person as I thought I was, that I don't deserve him, that I came to his daughter's wedding for the wrong reasons and with the wrong intentions. That I'm the phoniest Buddhist he'll ever meet. He'll hug me tight. He'll tell me that he loves me. He'll kiss my tears, ask me to fix myself and go back to the party with him; he'll remind me that he loves me as I wash my face, he'll say it again as I pat it dry and apply a new coat of mascara, as I put on my nylons and do my hair. And together, we'll make it back to the party, where I will smile into space looking ahead of me. Trying not to bump into Mary on the dance floor, trying not to pry open the back of the black dress she'll have changed into. Understanding that she has moved on and so should I, that my husband is not looking at her and longing for the past, that the music is fabulous, the estate is stunning, and nobody is judging me, nobody is talking about me, nobody cares. I will dance the night away, and slowly, in the time it takes a woman to study another woman's hair, I'll humbly accept the ultimate unknown known of my own insignificance.

Sonya Huber

Breathing

L ast night I woke up and lay in bed in the dark, and I noticed that my breath was even and smooth like a handblown glass vase. My mind couldn't wait to mess with that, so I paid attention a bit too aggressively and smashed the moment to jagged, hitching bits. I am a Buddhist who can't focus on the breath, and that's OK.

Thich Nhat Hahn's book *Peace Is Every Step* popped up on my college campus like the yellow dandelion on its cover as the First Gulf War raged. I wanted anything that said peace, and his sweet advice stuck with me: "Breathing in, I know I am breathing in. Breathing out, I smile." I liked the idea but felt it was written for another species. That year I slumped against walls, stretched out on floors, and lay on stretchers in various emergency rooms, not knowing yet that the mysterious death shroud was a panic attack—and another—and another. The anxiety snaked its tendrils upward and broke through my crust to pull me down, to make me stop. Where does it come from? Even that question is beside the point, born from roots in my family tree so complex that the living thing itself is like a baobab, the African tree with the amazing ability to send out new roots that reach the soil from each branch end. The structure of anxiety can be either a home or a cage; it is what it is.

Before I tell you what it feels like, promise me this: promise you won't say *Try yoga try massage try acupuncture try long walks try stress reduction.* I have tried and I do many of these things and more; I am ridiculously therapized and meditated. And on good days, I am serene. I get a little defensive at how hard I've tried to wrestle this sharp-edged jewel from my throat. Strangers want to help and all I want to do is sit and look at them, goggle-eyed, and recite the figure: all this personal solving costs money and time, and retreats and rests have felt scarce despite my blessings.

My throat chakra is all jacked up. A reiki master has held her hands above me, shared the images of blue whirlpools and hurricanes, tutted about my choking and constricted voice, realigned mysterious energies that later found themselves sliding again and again out of whack.

Briefly—because I don't want to trigger anyone else's implosion breathing—I will tell you that it feels like someone is wrapping a dark blanket around my head, and in the heat that catches in my ears and at my throat I feel my stomach and diaphragm muscles knitting in a clutch and refusing to work together. They seem to stair-step down, unwilling to descend, feeling their way as if following a narrow path down to a lava pit. I breathe fine when I'm not paying attention. Following some sort of personal Heisenberg uncertainty principle, the act of observing changes what's being observed.

During my first all-day meditation retreat at a Shambhala Center, I raised my hand in a sea of a hundred newbies and tried to describe the feeling to the teacher for the question-and-answer session. "It's like my breath grabs itself when I try to watch it," I said. "It's not smooth."

The teacher, who was very new to teaching and who seemed to be self-conscious, said he didn't know what I meant, that the only thing he'd experienced was a "little self-consciousness" in the first few minutes of meditation. I felt hopeless and remedial. At the next break, a woman sitting across the aisle stopped me as we got up from our cushions and said, "That happens to me too." We both shook our heads at our shared confusion but glad to have someone else to understand: it's that *thing.*

Sometime later that year, during another rare and precious all-day meditation retreat, I sat in a one-on-one question session with a Zen teacher in a room with large windows opening onto a south Georgia cypress swamp. In the midst of talking about something else, I admitted to her that it worked better for me to focus on my muscles, even on the thrum of my pulse, than on my breath. I was, askance, asking for a reaction or even a judgment.

She, in her shorn-head intelligence, simply nodded in encouragement. "Yes, do that. It doesn't matter. Whatever works for you." She told me she had noticed me sitting with rigidity and muscle tension. She said focusing on bodily sensations is a common and equally fruitful path in meditation, and that she thought it would help me in many ways. I exhaled, feeling for a moment just like any other meditation student, freed of my secret meditation training wheels, relieved that it could be productive to sidle up to the windpipe and glance at it in my peripheral vision.

That's what it feels like: I grip too tightly onto my own lungs, as I tend to grip at handholds and grasp at life. And this is a big part of meditation, too, noticing my grasping. In other words, for me, the breath is *not* the answer. I have to let it go. It's not the solution for me, and there is no cleansing magic carpet ride.

It's hard to know what another body feels like. Years of wondering about this specific ornate body and its mysteries and secrets has led me to doctors and diagnoses of rheumatoid arthritis and fibromyalgia. I don't even know how long I've been in pain because I don't remember a "before," and sometimes there's so much shit going on that it's hard to articulate that you're in actual physical pain on top of the mental headaches.

So it makes sense that the pain would also become part of the background, like white noise. It's as if I were trying to see my windpipe and only belatedly realized I was squinting through bead curtains and duffle bags and cardboard boxes in a dimly lit storage unit. The physical pain in my shoulders, hips, and hands are knots of tension that distract and drain my focus. But once I look at those bursts of pain directly, they dangle like beautiful challenging fruit, red and sweet and directly mine, that I can peel again and again. When I focus on the physical trouble spots, I feel such *relief.* I realize how tense I am, how afraid I am of being in pain. I'm one big wall of resistance to everything else going on in my body besides the breathing.

Just seeing that I'm a bag of bones and muscles and pain and, yes, also breathing is fantastic.

I found another hopeful nugget in *Shambhala: The Sacred Path of the Warrior*. Chögyam Trungpa Rinpoche writes that after an outbreath, "You simply come back to your posture, and you are ready for another outbreath. Go out and dissolve..." and "You have mind working with breath, but you always maintain body as a reference point." Elsewhere he writes that the bottom of every breath is a little death; that resonates so clearly with me. It's a leap to get from one breath to the next. That little death comforts me because it describes what I see from the bottom of the breath, looking down.

I turned forty last year. Mortality is a beautiful thing. This rough halfway point makes me feel like putting my hands on my hips and saying, *Holy hell, what a climb.* It's time to try less; the amount of effort required to get me to this moment has in some ways ensured that I would not be able to relax until I arrived. Everything in my jerry-rigged and duct-taped inventory got me here, away from certain rooms and places and people that spun my weathervane and tweaked my dials and levers. We are all strange and ornate; if I try to play amateur plumber and force open my problematic windpipe with a crowbar, I'm liable to break something else. Like anyone floating in samsara, I am not an equation that can be completely solved, because that is not the point. My gratitude has made me want to accept all these strange pieces and plumbing I have been given, including a psychically inflamed trachea with an attitude problem.

I hardly have panic attacks anymore; if one creeps up, it's part of the furniture instead of a monument to failure. I married a man with his own panic tendencies. That wasn't why I picked him, but it is a small part of our shared life and collectively it's no big deal. Through experience and the mysteries of the universe, we are both tuned to a frequency in which we hear the roar of worlds colliding. And they do. There's nothing inherently wrong with that or with us.

Part of why I love meditation is being able to watch my resistance and fear dissolve as I loosen my grip on "doing it right" and as I get beyond techniques and guiding images, like the Zen adage that a finger pointing at the moon is not the moon itself. There are moments where I know I'm breathing and don't care, like riding a bike with no hands, and it's golden. And it's a beautiful thing to sit next to a candle and be able to say, "Hi, heart. I feel you beating." My lungs are shy, but my heart is strong.

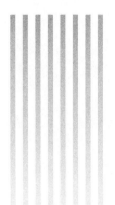

PART TWO

BALANCE

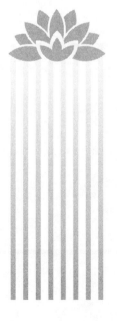

Dinty W. Moore

The Humpty Hatha

When the yoga teacher prompts us to extend our arms to reach the side walls, I sometimes extend mine until the shoulder muscles burn. When we're asked to twist and look at the back wall, I squeeze myself like a sponge. I'm a pretty stretchy soul, literally and figuratively, so give me a pose, any pose, and I can probably do it, or at least toss off an enthusiastic rendition. Yoga fits me well.

Unless I'm asked to balance.

Here's the problem: at fifty-something, I'm fairly overweight, and all of that extra poundage has settled uncomfortably into my middle-aged gut. The physics of this are not at all helpful when doing a Tree Pose, an Eagle, or the Warrior.

Imagine a small table with delicate legs, topped with forty or so hardcover books. The table inevitably wants to wobble and the books want very much to fall.

Or imagine Humpty Dumpty, up on that wall, trying to keep his center of gravity just so, lest he topple and break into shards of shell and yolk.

※ ※ ※

The unsteady egg serves as a pretty good metaphor for my life, on and off the mat. Those of us blessed enough to make it past the half-century mark know that day-to-day existence somehow becomes more not less complicated, though we had imagined it differently. I have a secure job, I have a stable marriage, I have a modest mutual fund account that might, just might if I'm lucky, allow me to retire someday, so shouldn't this daily riddle of living feel somehow less perplexing? I've conquered the demons of my youth, after all. I've acquired a little wisdom.

But no. I regularly struggle to balance life as a teacher, writer, husband, and parent with my life as an erratic yoga practitioner and caretaker of one wobbly, sagging human bundle of blood, flesh, and bone. How do I meet my obligations to others without ignoring the obligation to care for myself?

Often this boils down to the simple equation of finding ninety minutes on Monday afternoon to drag myself away from work and settle into yoga. Often, I even fail to do this.

※ ※ ※

Of course, my weight issues are about balance as well. I somehow can't find the proper equilibrium between wanting to eat magnificent food, to savor the pleasant sensation of taste and texture, the creativity of the culinary arts, with the necessity of stopping, limiting myself, exerting self-control.

So I am fat.

I hate saying that out loud—"I am fat"—but being honest with oneself is another form of balance, and one crucial lesson I've learned in my yoga practice is that all of life's balancing acts are, in the end, connected.

※ ※ ※

So I live an imbalance.

I like that term much better than *failure*. Imbalance is not so black-and-white, all-or-nothing. Rather than proposing a radical shift or an abysmal void, the word *imbalance* suggests that only a simple adjustment is needed. Like in the Tree Pose: that subtle shift of weight to center one's gravity.

But even small corrections can be daunting. In the yoga studio, teetering on one leg, I vacillate between gripping the floor with my five aching toes or, alternately, trying to release all tension from my body, to slip into alignment through relaxation and breath. One approach does not seem to support the other.

Outside of the studio I have my toe-gripping moments as well—stubbornness *can* be a virtue—and I have my moments of just taking a breath, dropping my shoulders, and feeling my way into the proper way to respond to a given situation.

The search for balance is never ending.

※ ※ ※

In yoga class the other day, attempting the Tree Pose with my back against the cold cinderblock wall, I was envying the skinny ones in the middle of the room, all straight-backed and steady. Heck, I told myself, if all I had above the waist were a few ribs, I could do this pose too. Better than them.

As if the point of it all was envy.

Or competition.

As if the point was to get the pose just right.

It struck me then:

"Your hand opens and closes, opens and closes," Rumi wrote. "If it were always a fist or always stretched open, you would be paralyzed."

How lucky I am to be teetering here.

How wonderful it is to be struggling for balance.

How fortunate if I could keep this skirmish going for fifty more years.

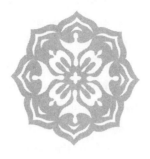

Neal Pollack

Yoga with My Dad

When you think of a "yogi," my dad isn't what comes to mind, unless you're thinking of Yogi Bear. Like me, he has excessive body hair and a preternatural fondness for luncheon meats. Unlike me, he's the son of immigrants who barely escaped Germany in 1934, and he served two tours of duty in Vietnam. Also, he watches Fox News at least three hours a day. But when I was in Phoenix for Thanksgiving, my dad and I went to a yoga class together.

Bernie has been taking morning yoga at his gym twice a week for two years. He considers it part of his workout routine. Sometimes he runs on the treadmill, sometimes he lifts weights, and sometimes he does yoga. "My trainer said it'd help my back," he told me.

"But there must be all kinds of other benefits," I said.

My dad, possessed of the least-troubled mind in existence, said, "Eh. I just feel good when it's done."

Usually, when I'm in Phoenix, I take yoga classes at a studio near my parents' house: expensive, sweaty numbers full of snotty people, pretentious flow, and overloud music of the type favored by new-money pseudospiritualists. The classes are at my physical level, sometimes even above. Therefore, I sweat acceptably, but I've never had a moment of decent conversation or authentic human connection during or after. Meanwhile, my dad goes off to yoga at the gym and arrives home calm and happy while I'm still sitting at the kitchen table in my boxers, staring glumly at my can of Diet Coke.

This time, I thought I'd try it his way. At dinner, I said, "Hey, Dad, will you take me to yoga tomorrow?"

He looked pleased, as though I'd asked if I could go to the office with him to see how he spent his day. But since I'd never actually asked for that, this was a fresh experience for both of us. It would be a genuine father–son outing.

"Of course," he said.

"Do you need a mat?" I asked. "I've got an extra in the car."

"I've got one," he said. "I've got two."

"Really? Where did you get them?"

"They sell them at TJ Maxx," my mom said.

The mainstreaming of yoga was complete.

My dad does his yoga in the workout room of a large chain fitness center near the intersection of Tatum and Shea, halfway between the Paradise Valley Mall and the Barry Goldwater Memorial. The aerobics steps and spinning cycles get moved to the side for the hour. Through the floor-to-ceiling rear glass wall, you can see dozens of people going through their morning workouts while watching *Fox and Friends*. But yoga cares not about politics and cares even less about notions of authenticity. This gym reminded me of where I'd begun my own practice, nearly eight years ago now.

My dad got to class almost fifteen minutes early. Just as I do, I thought. He put down his mat near the back left corner of the room. Just like me. He motioned for me to unroll my mat to his left.

"The other side's for Alice," he said.

"Who's Alice?" I asked.

"Oh, just someone who takes yoga," he said.

Aw, how cute, I thought. My dad has a yoga friend!

As it turned out, he had several, mostly around his age. The preclass conversation covered turkey and grandkids and college football, quite different from the conversations at my usual classes, which are usually about auditions and cats. By the time the teacher showed up, nearly fifty people had claimed their own yoga acre. There are definitely some challenges to teaching classes that size, but most of the teachers I know would stand on their heads for hours to get a class of four dozen people, because it would mean that they might actually be able to pay their rent through yoga.

The teacher carried a photo from the recent local Bikram-sponsored yoga championships, of which she's an aficionado. She showed it to a few students, who murmured that they'd never be able to do the pose shown in the picture. Other than the fact that she wore pink sweatpants with the word PURE written across the butt in black letters, this was the only thing for which I could criticize my dad's yoga teacher. Yoga isn't about perfecting poses. It's about living intelligently and kindly in the present moment. Poses, whatever the result, are just a by-product of the effort and concentration you put into them.

But once the class started, she said pretty much the same thing: having people focus on their breath, calling yoga a "beautiful gift," leading her mostly late-Boomer crowd through a slow, mindful flow, respectful of their needs and not condescending to them. I made a conscious effort to mind my own practice and not care about what was going on around me. At one point, though, I glanced at my dad. He was rolling on his back, knees drawn to his chest, with a look of extreme pleasure on his face like a dog getting its belly rubbed.

I didn't ever want to see that again.

The only other time I became aware of him was when the teacher called for Bow Pose, and dad said, "I don't do that one." That's a very excusable admission for a man who's had rotator-cuff surgery and who once broke his shoulder in a skiing accident. He doesn't need to do Bow Pose.

When the teacher said *namaste* after a short Savasana, most of the class applauded. I've taken yoga classes all over the world, from a great variety of master teachers. Rarely have I heard such enthusiasm. These people were never going to attend an Anusara Grand Gathering or Wanderlust, buy tickets to a "trance dance," or download an MC Yogi song. They probably didn't know, and probably didn't care, about the difference between Ashtanga, Iyengar, or kundalini yoga. None of them would sign up as Lululemon ambassadors. But they'd arrived that day at the gym stiff, or feeling stressed out, or bloated from Thanksgiving dinner, and now they were a little better. Yoga serves no more important purpose. The rest of what we call "yoga" in the West is often just sickly-sweet frosting atop a delicious cake that needs no extra flavor.

Then the 9:45 aerobics people came barging in, as they're wont to do during gym yoga, and the spell broke. My dad and I drove home, sipping on our Costco plastic water bottles that he keeps cold in the garage mini-fridge.

"So, was that different than usual?" I asked him.

"Eh, maybe a little more rushed," he said. "Big class because of the holidays. Good, though."

"How was the class for you?"

"I can do some of the poses," he said. "Some of the poses, I can't do. It's fine for me."

My dad, the yogi.

Amy Monticello

Against the Pursuit of Happiness: A Meditation

Listen. Happiness? It just looks different on people like me.

—LIDIA YUKNAVITCH,
THE CHRONOLOGY OF WATER

In Ithaca, New York, Tibetan prayer flags hang from the eaves of rambling Victorian houses, and quaint little carriage houses, and dilapidated A-frame houses with Pabst beer cans lining porch railings. Their lilting red, blue, orange, white, and yellow squares make no sound in the breeze, so thin and soft is the translucent fabric. On Aurora Street, in Ithaca's Fall Creek neighborhood, the Namgyal

Monastery Institute of Buddhist Studies sits nestled in a nonde-script turn-of-the-twentieth-century house painted a deep burgundy with gold trim. The prayer flags light up the house like year-round Christmas decorations. Down the narrow alleyway running just behind the monastery, Cascadilla Creek burbles over shalestone, plastic bottles, discarded road signs, and outposts of tall, thick grasses that curve like spider plants.

When I walk my dog daily past the monastery, I sometimes glimpse Namgyal's monks, their maroon or orange robes shushing as they slowly walk the neighborhood, or work in the small front garden, or mow the lawn with a quiet push mower. My pup, a high-strung cattle dog mix, sniffs the short trains of the robes suspiciously, takes a few steps sideways. Then she pulls me down the alley toward home.

If you're from anywhere else in upstate New York, Ithaca seems as mythic as its Homeric namesake. My friend Vini actually calls the city "Mythaca." We laugh about this on coffee dates, where we also discuss her therapy appointments and my ongoing struggle with generalized anxiety disorder. We poke gentle fun at the former flower children who wear Flax linen clothes and take three kinds of yoga classes. Vini and I both wear a lot of black and rely on tennis and cycling, respec-tively, to manage stress.

And like Odysseus's home, the one to which he can never really return after the Trojan War, Ithaca is sensationalized, a cari-cature of itself. Even the graffiti is Ithaca brand. On the wall of the former library, before the city commissioned a vibrant mural, a tag artist kept spray-painting the word RESPECT on the stucco wall. BE HAPPY reads the sidewalk on Linn Street.

In homage to the glacial lakes, waterfalls, and gorges that make up Ithaca's abundant natural wonders, you can buy a T-shirt emblazoned with ITHACA IS GORGES. I'm a bigger fan of its variant: ITHACA IS COLD.

A popular bumper sticker here reads ITHACA: TEN SQUARE MILES SURROUNDED BY REALITY.

The city boasts an economy buoyed by the presence of Cornell University and Ithaca College, my alma mater. Unlike other postindustrial places in upstate New York, cities like Binghamton, Syracuse, and Utica—virtual economic and artistic deserts—Ithaca has an art theater, an independent bookstore co-owned by members of the community, a long list of thriving restaurants that use locally sourced ingredients, and a public dog park democratically designed with sections for small and large dogs.

I grew up in greater Binghamton, about an hour south of Ithaca. The area was once home to the Endicott-Johnson shoe factory, and later, the IBM corporation, but now it claims record unemployment, perpetually gray skies, and structural damage from two massive floods that struck five years apart. In March 2012, just months after the second floodwaters receded, Gallup released its annual quality-of-life polls, and Binghamton's scores reflected its dismal state: #1 in most pessimistic, #5 in most depressed, and #2 in most obese nationwide. My mother emailed me the newspaper article, complete with a comments section suggesting that Binghamton residents took a slanted sort of pride in these designations—their worries and heartaches, their cynicism and lack of ambition, their waists and butts, all justified by the extremity of their living conditions. The pervading attitude was, like, "Yeah, we're fat and think most things suck, but we're still here, and that makes us way more badass than you." I laughed. And I felt a little homesick, to tell the truth. I kind of like being extreme. I kind of like being sad.

❀ ❀ ❀

I've always been conflicted about the pursuit-of-happiness line in the Declaration of Independence. On the one hand, it's a hopeful and ballsy move on the part of the taxed-without-representation colonists. On the other hand, I detect arrogance at the core of Jefferson's ideal.

I'm not well versed on the philosophies of the Enlightenment, so I can only talk about this from a personal and contemporary perspective, and how I believe Western (OK, American) sensibilities about happiness are corrupting, or at least changing, Eastern practices of yoga and meditation now championed in every remotely progressive pocket of the nation. The population of Ithaca hovers around 35,000, which classifies it as a small city, but residents can choose between over twenty different yoga studios advertised in our White Pages. In addition to the Namgyal Monastery, we also have the Zen Center, a sixty-acre facility formed from the dregs of an old hippie commune. Both Cornell University and Ithaca College offer meditation classes for credit, and yoga and Pilates classes run daily at their fitness centers. The majority of my friends and colleagues can make enthusiastic recommendations about where to go for the Ashtanga, Bikram, Iyengar, Kripalu, Sivananda, hot, power, restorative, or children's yoga to which they're most loyal.

One colleague, when contemplating whether or not to move

from the area, said, "I already have a yoga class here. I'm settled."

I'm being hard on Ithaca, flippant toward its healthy sense of self, but the fact is, I went to college here, left for graduate school and my first teaching job, and then returned to teach at my alma mater when I could no longer take living in rural Alabama. I love it here. I love the gorges slicing through the city like ancient Roman aqueducts. I love the paper-scented independent bookstore and the inky-dark art theater. I love the smorgasbord of yoga studios with their tall, sun-drenched windows and shiny, blond-wood floors. I love the optimistic graffiti and happy, Flax-clad people.

But back when I was in college—when I was in the reckoning of woman-daughter-writer—sometimes my anger at Ithaca's relentless optimism won out over my love for its good heart. And sometimes I wanted to run down my yoga-practicing, meditating boyfriend in my car.

Let's call him Simon. Simon, who tried to save me.

If anyone has ever tried to save you, then you know how infuriating it is. How there's arrogance at the core of that, too.

Simon and I dated for three mostly turbulent years. I was an atheist substance-abusing writer, and he was a secularist-Taoist-Buddhist occasionally substance-abusing writer. We fought constantly. Standing barefoot in the street fighting. Drunken phone call fighting. Slamming doors and punching walls fighting. I admit most of it was my fault. Simon would say things like I needed to be happier, and I resented him for it. Like other young, financially independent women discovering the inequities of gendered life amid creative writing and women's studies classes, I felt entitled to my rage. Obligated, even. Rage was my feminist cause.

In his last semester in college, Simon took a meditation class as an elective. The class was taught by the Jewish rabbi who ran the multifaith chapel on campus. Simon, who had pronounced attention deficit disorder, eventually passed a final exam delivered in the form of a twelve-hour silent meditation. I realize now what an accomplishment this was.

I didn't take the class, but I hated it anyway. Simon became obsessed with meditation. He meditated in the middle of parties. He meditated while driving. He meditated at the gym while I ran myself into a frenzied sweat. I'm exaggerating some of this. But what's true is that Simon was discovering his serenity and silence at the same time I was discovering my anger and voice.

Simon tried to teach me meditation as a cure for the vicious insomnia that dominated my college years with its static gray chokehold. At night, when I lay awake in bed clenching my leg and jaw muscles, a fierce shadow spreading over my electric and exhausted insides, Simon told me to banish my thoughts and focus on my breath. Most nights, I ended up banishing him from my apartment. Then I stayed up all night listening to Carissa's Wierd (the band's spelling) and talking softly aloud to the white cabinet that hung in the corner of my room.

Simon bugged me for months to go with him to Namgyal, where the exiled Tibetan monks offered free public meditation three evenings a week. When I finally agreed on a snowy winter night—crisp and clear and brick cold—I focused so hard on my breathing that I ended up hyperventilating on the floor cushions.

AMY MONTICELLO

The conflation of meditative practices (and "meditative," in this sense, refers to sustained contemplation and reflection, as well as yogic posing, transcendental chanting, and other religious forms of meditation) with increased levels of happiness seems to be a uniquely Western notion. To be "Zen" in the West is to not let shit get you down. Not to be unmoored by negative emotions, or to dismiss them. Americans in particular have become uncomfortable with feelings of depression, anxiety, anger, loneliness, and jealousy. Buddhist meditation stresses the confrontation and release of suffering; the concept of happiness in most Buddhist cultures is called Enlightenment, which is something more akin to powerful, resourceful self-awareness. But for Americans, feelings of suffering symbolize a failure at our own pursuits of happiness. To feel unhappy is unpatriotic.

Several years ago, on the advice of my doctor in Alabama, I began taking an antidepressant to cope with the sizable depression that came with isolation in a place far from my home. My grandfather had just died, and my father had had his first heart attack. I felt helpless and despairing, over eleven hundred miles away from Ithaca, in a house surrounded by acres of cow pastures and no people. My husband was proud of me for taking a calculated step toward feeling better. But I was embarrassed by my decision. My mother has taken Prozac for two decades, and I associated meds with hitting an emotional bankruptcy I hoped never to see myself.

My fears were confirmed when I confessed to a lifelong friend about my new prescription. Let's call her Karen.

Karen and I were in her car, on our way to go hiking during

one of my breaks from teaching, when I told her I had started taking Pristiq. "Figures," she said darkly, taking a sip of coffee from her thermos.

"Figures what?" I said.

"Figures you'd choose a pill over choosing happiness. Why can't you just choose happiness?"

In February 2012, the formidable online journal *Slate* reported that "impatience trounces sympathy" for Facebook users reading others' negative status updates. Citing a study from the University of Waterloo, Katy Waldman found that more self-confident Facebook users have less tolerance for others' use of the social networking site as a "safe space" for sharing sans cheerful lacquer. "I find these results oddly heartbreaking," writes Waldman. "It seems an irony typical of the Internet that the people who feel safest expressing themselves online actually damage their social standing when they do so. Not because they're somehow opting out of the real world, as Facebook critics like to insist, but because they are lulled into relaxing their façades."

Recently, I polled my Facebook friends about depression and anxiety. How does it manifest, I asked? How does it affect their loved ones? Their work? Their public personas? I was floored by the responses. First, they were largely categorical. In general, men reported worrying over money and job security, and tended to make jokes that included six-packs as coping mechanisms (both the literal and figurative kinds of six-packs). On the other hand, women mostly reported worrying about worrying itself. The notion that they may not be as happy as other people distressed them, and this fear became a secret they carried just under the surface of their grateful, glowing Facebook statuses and pictures of their kids' birthday parties, like "a volcanic hot spot," as one responder put it, something that would, she thought, inevitably get expressed.

How did they express it?

In a deluge of private messages, these women revealed the true nature of their anxiety and depression. They drink. They save answering machine messages in case it's the last time they hear someone's voice. They close their eyes before making a left-hand turn in their cars. They put their psychotropic drugs in Tic-Tac containers. They check into hospitals with their vacation time so their coworkers won't know where they are.

I cried while reading one of the messages. It came from the wife of one of my dearest friends. She and her husband are devout Christians with two beautiful daughters, a New England home close to family, and what appears on Facebook to be hundreds of loving friends. For years, I've admired her photo albums (she's a talented and prolific photographer), quaking a little at the sight of so much centrality of family, so much happiness. What I didn't see—what no one saw—was my friend's wife cutting herself alone in the bathroom.

At the time of our conversation about my antidepressants, Karen had been practicing yoga regularly for years. I took her callousness seriously, took for granted that her lifestyle meant she knew more than me about what it takes to be happy. Shortly after our hike that day, I quit taking the pills. I'll never know if or how they would have helped.

But something else happened around that time, too. I went inward and started writing again. To be economical about this, I'll just say it turns out that the best writing comes from an empathic place. A place that can vividly imagine another's experience of life without judging that experience, without otherizing it. And that empathy—its daily practice—can be quite meditative in its own right. It can even bring its practitioner something like peace. Something like joy.

※ ※ ※

Today, some aspects of the American pursuit of happiness are built precisely in place of empathy. Jeffrey Sachs, writing for the *Huffington Post*, claims that corporate policies like the ones that have left the majority of upstate New York financially crushed have created "the logic of America, to the point that the Supreme Court can no longer tell the difference between free speech and untrammeled corporate power." And such corporate domination of our politics and media, Sachs believes, has left Americans with a dearth of "trust, honesty, and compassion."

It's no wonder, then, that Binghamton is pessimistic, depressed, and gaining weight.

But Sachs also describes a country he sees as the globe's great hope. In the tiny Himalayan country of Bhutan, Prime Minister Jigme Thinley has developed what he calls Gross National Happiness (as opposed to gross national product). Together with Sachs, Thinley hosted a congregation of world leaders to discuss how individual countries can begin to reprioritize national efforts so as to better support "a sense of community, trust, and environmental sustainability." Unsurprisingly, all three require more empathic economic philosophies. With an emphasis on meeting people's basic needs (which the author identifies as clean water, health care, education, and "meaningful" employment), striking a balance between healthy consumerism and healthy living, preserving the planet's natural viability, and developing more nuanced systems for measuring a society's well-being, Sachs and Thinley believe we can raise the global happiness quotient.

Such conferences do indeed spark optimism in me. In fact, descriptions of this utopian world society sound a bit familiar.

They sound like Mythaca.

☙ ❧ ☙

There I go again, getting snide. Let me bring this meditation on happiness back to its breath: language.

Part of my resistance to the Zen culture of America comes from the way we narrowly and simplistically define its terms. Happiness should be devoid of sadness. Meditation should be quiet. Yoga should be done on a mat in a bright room. Though I respect that studied masters of these practices have developed systems to help people achieve their well-being goals, I think it's time we allowed for other interpretations of what is yogic, meditative, or happy.

For example, I just saw a post on Facebook—a picture of a snowy road with the words "Quietest people have the loudest minds" printed across the top. The sentiment suggests that quiet people think more deeply or actively than talkative people. If this is the case, then I'm intellectually screwed.

I'm a loud person. I've been told by family, friends, and colleagues that my voice "carries." Meaning that if you listened to a group of people on tape, you can pick out my voice immediately. It's not because I'm trying to drown other people out, but because I take solace in using my voice. I use it to move more comfortably through the world. This is as true in writing as it is in speech.

My husband jokes that he can always tell when I'm working on an essay because I'll talk at him, not with him. "You're talking your way to meaning," he says. "You have to vocalize your understanding before it's real to you." He loves me, so he listens generously to the one-woman show playing weekly at our house.

When we lived in Alabama surrounded by cow pastures and no people, I thought I was going to die of silence. Our house was set back so far from the road I couldn't even hear the logging trucks go by. During the day, when I'd step outside to let the dog run around, I'd feel my chest tighten with every second of silence that encroached on me. That's how my anxiety works: at night, before bed, in remote, peopleless spaces, after too much time in literary isolation, anxiety comes and steals my breath.

I fall asleep with the TV on. I feel at ease in New York City.

I'm also a cardioholic. While Simon was trying to teach me how to regulate my breathing through meditation, I was teaching myself how to regulate my heartbeat through cardio exercise. In college, I attracted the stares of many a gym bunny for the way I ran on the treadmill, pumped on the elliptical, climbed on the Stairmaster. I sweat hard. My ponytailed hair does not look cute. There is such freedom in not looking cute while exercising in mixed company.

Lately, I'm addicted to spinning, a form of intense indoor cycling offered at my gym. A yoga class meets across the hall from the cycling room, and my instructor, a triathlete, often refers to our class as anti-yoga. It makes us laugh and taps into the cyclist's desire to be something closer to Binghamton-style hardcore, but really, I think the comparison is less justified than we'd like to believe. In spinning, we work on form and endurance in our "poses." There's the seated flat, with arrow pose. There's the standing climb pose. There's the jogging pose, fingertips lightly resting on the flat of the handlebars. Sometimes we work on "quieting" our upper bodies and concentrating solely on moving our legs. Sometimes we use only our right leg to pedal. Then our left. With each pose, the goal is to sustain—our heart rates, our resistance levels, our postures, and our mental clarity to endure.

When I get restless or short-tempered at home, my husband never asks about my menstrual cycle. He asks about the last time I went to the gym.

I have been back to Namgyal, though. My friend Katie and I started going to the monastery's public meditation on Wednesdays this summer. For me, it was part research. But I made a promise to myself not to get hung up on meditating "correctly." Instead, I would meditate however it felt best.

Going back to the monastery allowed me a better look at the significance of asylum. Founded in 1992, Namgyal provides shelter for the exiled Tibetan monks who live there, which means that Ithaca's empathy has literally saved their spiritual lives. Here, they can practice and teach and live peaceably.

The meditation room, located on the first floor in what would traditionally be someone's living room, has about twenty blue mats and circular cushions for the public to use. The monks who lead the meditation sit at the front of the room, off to the side in front of the fireplace. The displays on the mantel and in the open facing cabinets and shelves are curious. Stacked cans of Bumblebee tuna. Planters peanuts. Del Monte fruit cocktail. An Ithaca College graduation medal draped over a light fixture. A row of figurines that look like Tibetan versions of Hummels. A vase of fake flowers.

The meditation sessions last approximately forty-five minutes. They start and finish with Tibetan chanting, performed in rumbling, gravelly tones. In the middle there is about twenty minutes of silent meditation. The monks never address us in English, or give us instructions on what to do with our legs and arms and breath. They simply begin.

※ ※ ※

My friend Marissa, a writer and yoga teacher, occupies a special place in my heart. She, too, once lived in Mythaca with me, and describes herself as doggedly optimistic. But the writer in her reaches for me across the divide of our differences, and vice versa. When I'm sad—and like a good Binghamton native, I'm prone to sadness and pessimism, if not obesity—Marissa never tells me to buck up and go to yoga class. She encourages me to write. She is intimate with writing's meditative qualities. She knows how writing sustains.

In turn, I listen when she tells me that, just as people judge me as unhappy, people judge her as naïve. Apparently, to feel anything too openly in our culture is to invite suspicion.

Marissa told me something really beautiful once, something that galvanized East and West. She said that her favorite part of yoga class is the final relaxation pose. "Sometimes," she said, "I just collapse on the mat and burst into tears."

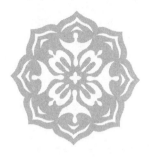

Elizabeth Kadetsky

Swerve

Gina and our mother have this game. They stand at opposite ends of my mother's apartment tossing a super ball to each other and watching the cat, Cookie, chase it from the bedroom straight on through to the kitchen. This is especially fun because it's a railroad flat—four rooms strung together like carts on a track. Cookie runs back and forth. Again and again. No one ever gets tired of this—until Gina does.

I'm watching the three of them do this and thinking of my student with the wandering eye last week hula-waving her eyes over to the side, along with her hands. Her two eyes stared off into an invisible distance or distances, as she used the word *swerve* to describe the technique in a short story we read in class. A swerve side-winds the reader when it surfaces in a last, careen-to-the-side-of-the-highway paragraph. The swerve is a relevant but different story, taking place on the shoulder of the road where you were too distracted to look for a real story.

This looking in the wrong place is also a kind of *viparyaya*, or error, I am thinking now as I watch the ball, followed by the cat, ricochet from one end to the other of the flat. The swerve might even be an error of a higher phylum, such as *avidya*—misconception, or delusion. Swerve, *viparyaya*, *avidya*, I go on thinking and tuning out. *Viparyaya,* from Patañjali yoga, means delusion and basically suggests that it is impossible to see anything clearly unless one has stripped away all the veils of prejudice, hope, worry, traumatic memory, wishful thinking, and projection that clutter everyday experience. Then one is yogically enlightened. Until then, one is blinded by this tendency to think the real problem lies elsewhere when in fact it's directly in front of you, goading.

My mother loves me after all, for instance, even if she could never remember a damned thing about me. *I'm a vegetarian. I teach at Penn State and move out there from New York City for the semesters fall and spring. My ex and I broke up. If there's chicken in the ramen I don't eat it.* Now that we know memory was the problem and nothing passive aggressive, we also know that our mother will die. This awful disease will take her. *Swerve.*

Gina takes care of our mother in exchange for free room and board with her at the flat, in Long Island City, and a small stipend from our mother's retirement account. My contribution, since I have an actual job, is to repair the small things, which are increasingly transforming to big things. It feels good to fix tangible problems when I can't staunch the mortal ones: atrophy, decay, slow death. My other duty is to spend several hours a week on the phone with Gina talking her down from crises.

Today: my mother didn't want to wash her hair. This is the problem I'm focused on now. I have brought fancy shampoos. Where's the swerve, I think, as I unpack the pleasingly shaped bottles onto the kitchen table while Gina watches and giggles. Is it the hair? Like any swerve, I'll never see it or else it wouldn't be a swerve. "Doesn't this smell *nice*?" I say to our mother while scowling at Gina.

My mother sniffs one and gets an abstracted expression, concentrating hard. "*Lovely*! Oh, Suezy, that is really nice. Peaches," she says.

✻ ✻ ✻

After the memory problem and before the hair, my mind was on an overbearing social worker I call Miss Malaprop. She had been phoning to tell me our mother would get lost if we left her at home alone or let her go out—"not that she's a prisoner or anything."

Our mother is a "wander risk." She likes to go walking—walking and walking, miles a day. Alzheimer's and wandering turn out to be closely associated. Six months ago she went out and didn't come home. I called the cops and they found her at 3:00 a.m. aimlessly exploring the nearby housing projects beneath the Fifty-ninth Street bridge.

This was when Malaprop insisted we increase our surveillance. I told her it wasn't possible to increase Gina's already burdensome commitment to the project of keeping our mother busy, so Malaprop agreed to help us out with the 24/7 situation by receiving our mother at her adult day-care center every morning—paid for by Medicaid—from 7:00 a.m. until the van dropped her off at home, anytime between one and three in the afternoon. Problem: solved.

This was good, because Gina is going crazy. She's no good with stress, and the living here exacerbates chronic back pain that makes it impossible for her to hold a job and often makes her depressed and immobile. There is a well-known condition called caregiver's dementia. The Alzheimer's Association reports that more than 33 percent of family caregivers report symptoms of depression. Caregivers are mostly women. Our compassion will kill us. Gina often sends me text messages with signoffs such as *Love, your psychologically very fragile sister Gina*. So, I am relieved that Malaprop has offered up this activity to occupy our mother's daytimes.

For a brief respite, many obstacles seem to clear. The hair crisis averted, I go to yoga and accomplish Galavasana to Sirsasana to Chaturanga. This includes an arm balance, and a headstand, and a thrilling leap through the air. I feel mastery. My body glides through space; I control each minuscule muscle movement. In the class, Frank, the teacher, says, "When it's about ninety-eight-point-six degrees like this I feel like the air is meeting me, it's hugging me." I also believe that the universe is coming to meet me; it is watching out for me and my small family.

Later that day, Malaprop phones. "How are you, Elizabeth,

how are you?" She is calling to deliver the next swerve. Malaprop is Malaprop because she speaks in clichés.

"Fine, thanks, Malaprop. How are you?" Actually, I call her by her real name. Malaprop likes to say my name so much, I offer hers as often as possible as well.

"Not so good, Elizabeth, not so good. The van has been waiting to drop off your mom for an hour and a half, Elizabeth. An hour and a half."

I'm in my apartment in the East Village, and the van brings my mother to her apartment twenty minutes away from me near the Vernon/Jackson stop on the 7. The tradeoff for daily day care is that someone must be waiting at her flat on Vernon Boulevard when the center sends our mother home. She has been brought home in the van, but Gina is not there to receive her, is what Malaprop is saying. Gina said she'd be. I meet the van sometimes too, but not today.

"Elizabeth, you know we've had this problem before, Elizabeth." The van has not been able to drop off my mother today because no one is there to receive her. My mother and the van driver have been waiting on the sidewalk an hour and a half. The driver keeps buzzing upstairs for Gina but no one answers. Gina has missed the van drop-off a dozen times already. Malaprop makes each of these statements three times.

They're cutting us off, Malaprop adds. *Swerve.* This statement startles me so much I ignore it. They're kicking our mother out of the day program, Malaprop repeats, because Gina has missed the van too many times. Malaprop repeats her statement a third time, and then a fourth and fifth, such that I can no longer ignore it. I recognize that a new order of problem has entered.

❧ ❧ ❧

On the other hand, by the time I get off the subway on Vernon twenty minutes later, my mind has moved past the current obstacle and projected itself to the next one. I aim to complete an A/C installation that I began last week but couldn't finish because it turned out the socket was busted. I have a power strip to attach the new unit to a working outlet; foam to weather-strip it; blue tape to cover the burned electrical plate. I'm not thinking of the inevitable swerve really—for instance, where is Gina?

It's the hottest day of the year so far. I can make out my mother from the subway exit two blocks away, dressed in white and spreading her arms at me and doing one of her dances. Up into her forties she supported us as a working fashion model, and though she is seventy-one now, people generally think she's fifty. Her hair is thick and black, her face expressive, olive skinned, dramatic. She remains a beautiful woman.

"Aren't you hot?" I ask when I reach her.

She hugs me. "It's so nice to see you, my darling! Look at you. Your hair! What did you do? Your teeth! They're so…great! Just great!" There is also pantomime, gesture, Japanese Noh theater. She spins me around, looks, hugs again.

"Aren't you hot?" I repeat. The heat is making me dazed.

"I don't mind the heat." It's rising off the pavement in ripply patterns. She hugs the van driver, who is visibly sweating from open pores on his reddened forehead, nose and cheeks.

"Your mother is very nice lady," he says, in his accent, in spite of the two hours.

My mother and I walk up the stairs to her third-floor landing, and I think about how it's fortuitous I made it out to Long Island City for this hottest day of the year so Gina and my mother can have A/C. I'm not thinking of the inevitable swerve, though as my mother walks ahead of me on the steps I do think to ring Malaprop to beg for a reprieve. My mother can't actually be kicked out from the seven-day-a-week program. Then what would we do? It's unthinkable.

Malaprop starts right in when she picks up, as if there has been no interruption of time or distance or mental distraction since our last chat. "It's more times than we realized, Elizabeth. The van company thought they could work directly with the client themselves, which I didn't know about, and now the normal procedure—"

Malaprop's voice drones on as I reach the inside of the flat with my mother trailing behind and walk into the bedroom to deposit the A/C supplies. There, I am startled by the sight of Gina passed out on her bed.

Swerve.

I hang up on Malaprop. Just like that. *Click.* And she's gone.

Gina has cut marks and thin patches of dry blood on one arm. The blood is cracked and translucent, not copious, not like she slit her wrist or anything... *Or anything.*

I call David, Gina's therapist, to tell him there's an emergency. I leave a message.

I don't think Gina's body is a corpse. I think, *She's not dead.* I think that I can see, barely, a small movement in her chest. Rather,

I imagine what it would be like if she were a corpse. I am vaguely aware of my mother standing behind me peering at Gina from over my shoulder. I see two images of Gina in parallax: one as she is, the other as a corpse. Slowly, slowly, the two images move closer together until they're lined up. Then I realize there's virtually no difference.

I experience the moving of adrenaline through me as a pulse. I walk to the bed. My mother is behind me mirroring each of my steps. Things could go either way. I put my hand on Gina's shoulder and rock her a little. My mind is also on Malaprop and the no-day-center problem, and the air conditioner and the supplies to install, which still dangle from my hand in their plastic bag. Wherever the swerve might be, I continue to believe in a small part of me that I have arrived at the apartment prepared for it. Also, I feel I am not really in the room but somewhere else, or maybe up in the corner.

Gina doesn't wake up, but she's breathing.

I shake harder and her eyes slit open.

"Do I need to call an ambulance?" I ask her.

"*Noooo*," she moans. "I'm just tired. Really, really tired." She nods back out.

I wake her again. "What are the cuts?"

"I broke a glass in the sink while I was doing dishes. Leave me alone. You don't understand. You never understand."

"Understand what?"

She passes out again.

I wake her again. "You missed the van. They were buzzing and buzzing."

She pops up to sitting. "What time is it? Oh no!" Then she conks right back out.

My mother stands beside me peering at Gina and then looking back to me while affecting empathic faces. She pantomimes concern, looks at Gina with the same mime expression, then makes an exaggerated *Poor baby* pout, and addresses it to me, then to Gina, then to me. I realize she has no idea what's going on. I nonetheless try to reassure her by acting as if everything's under control.

My gesture may be empty too, but its effect is real, at least on me. I wonder if this would be different if I were alone. I wonder if I *am* alone. I didn't understand, Gina was right about that. My mother has been playing a role that looks like being present, and so I have been reading her as present.

She gets right into her bed and pulls up her covers to below her chin and smiles at me and begins to watch me as if I am a TV, with an expression of amused curiosity and intrigue. From the bed parallel to hers, Gina blearily comes to consciousness and observes me too.

As if this is another of the most normal afternoons of the year, without thinking really, I work on the A/C install with the foam strips and weatherproofing tape. My mind is still on the problems. It has not caught up with the swerve yet. The socket is ringed in soot, so I cover it with a sign and the blue tape—DO NOT TOUCH. Then I attach the power cord to a plug at the far end of the room and turn on the A/C. It is huge—14,000 BTUs—and I put it on 60 degrees and the highest fan setting.

This instantly blows the reset button on the new power strip. I set it again and lower the fan, and now it keeps running. It seems to do little to cool the room, but Gina and my mother are sleeping and dozing as if they're fine.

Looking back, I remember how there was a time lag between my perception of circumstances and my reaction. For that second, when she was lying there on that bed, Gina looked to me like a corpse. What would I have done? Now, I think, *Did I actually do this?*

I was operating according to *Hotel Rwanda* logic. You think you have hit bottom and then you're taken another notch lower, but you're still operating according to the idea that the old floor is your bottom. One death stuns you and then suddenly there is mass murder. I tell my students to watch *Hotel Rwanda* to learn structure. A swerve, I tell them, creates surprise and reversal and moves the plot.

The next morning in my apartment I wake up to the reality that, unlike every other day for the past several weeks, now my mother has no day program to attend because Malaprop has kicked her out. I'd been trying to line up extra care to lessen Gina's afternoon hours. I was trying to solve the problem that there wasn't enough daytime care; now I must confront the reality that there's even less. My new struggle is to recoup what we had.

David has returned my call and told me that he recommends Gina admit herself to the psych unit at Bellevue, and Gina has texted to say she's going.

I should have been more compassionate. I call Gina and tell her that I agree with David and that she should go. We'll manage without her, of course, I say.

I make a list of people to call and one by one start leaving messages.

I'm still in bed. I make another list:

Don't make phone calls from bed.

Don't make them in hundred-degree heat walking down the sidewalk.

Don't give in to crisis thinking.

One crisis need not snowball to the next.

Every present moment exists in its own time.

The trauma of the present moment needn't infect the moment that follows.

Then I look up a saying that I read recently in a compendium of Buddhist aphorisms about how panic doesn't help:

"Do not encumber your mind with useless thoughts. What good does it do to brood on the past or anticipate the future?"

—DILGO KHYENTSE RINPOCHE

I make an appointment at a new day center off Queens Boulevard where my mother could possibly start, though they don't take Medicaid, and walk to the Union Square subway feeling in control nonetheless. I am in my body, as if floating, lithe and in the air. *I will function, I will fly.* I think of the feeling in yoga yesterday. *I pulsed through the air.* The heat is already pressing down on me, and I think of what Frank said. *The air is meeting me.* The yogis are relentless bright-siders; Gina has always hated this about me.

On the subway out to the community center, I write more

reminders-to-self in my notebook: *Be in the moment. Observe the flickering present. Hone perception. Act in the instant.* Another yoga teacher, Cyndi, recently recommended subscribing to a daily cell-phone widget from Swami Satchidananda. "They say really wise things," she said, "like, *Don't worry. It doesn't actually help.*" I add this wisdom to my list.

And then the train hits the elevated rail tracks above Queens Boulevard, and I move into cell phone reception and the phone rings, and I answer, and all my resolutions are to naught. I depart the station on Queens Boulevard and Fortieth Street with the phone already attached to my ear. I am wandering in the unmitigated heat and glare, lost on the hot pavement in Queens, just as forecasted. Since I don't know where I'm going and can't use the GPS on my phone while I'm using it, I sit on the sidewalk. Now I'm talking in hundred-degree heat on the pavement.

It is Sue, from an affordable home-care agency that has already sent us a low-cost aide, Veta, for twelve hours a week. We can barely afford Veta, but I've called Sue to ask for another Veta.

"It takes me minimum two weeks to do a search," Sue tells me.

"I really can't talk because we're in a crisis and I have to find someone right now."

"Let me just give you two numbers, two numbers"—and she gives me numbers for two emergency home-care agencies, which before hanging up on her I write down on a slip of paper that I promptly lose.

Before I put it away my phone rings again. It is David. He says that he believes Gina's attempt to take her life "wasn't serious."

"She was attempting to take her life?" *I knew this, didn't I?*

Swerve.

He doesn't want her to try again, he's saying. Gina should get into the psych ward. They want me to come to an 11:00 a.m. meeting.

"I can't. I can't take care of everybody."

"Yes it's not an ideal world, and in an ideal world you could come."

⁂

I move in with my mother. There are no other options. I wish the circumstances had something to do with me, some failing—me, a child-woman, seeking the succor of a welcoming parent. I would come to heal myself with maternal nurturing after a tough trial in the world out there, with a man, or a job—maybe drugs or an illness. Perhaps the world got too rough for me. The universe was unkind to me. But there was never that out. My failing was being able. When everyone else falls down, I show up to catch them.

The hard part is the not sleeping. Starting at 5:00 a.m., my mother is walking around my bed in a semicircle talking to herself—*Who is she? What's she doing here?* I slide down my facemask, smile, say, *It's me, Lizzy, your daughter,* and her face relaxes from fear to relief. *Oh, good. Phew.*

I get in a routine where, when Veta comes, I bike across the river to my apartment to pick up clothes and go to yoga classes. On the bridge I feel the openness of river and sky. Life feels like life—*living*—not so much a problem as an adventure. I feel hyperacute and present. I start to think of my days at my mother's as my job for now, and in fact

I start to like it. I think I'm good at it, coming up with activities—art therapy, drawing in the park, speed-walking to burn off energy.

"*The obstacle is the path*," reads another aphorism in my Buddhist compendium. My mother is who she is. Giddy half the time, despairing the other. Chattering. She is full of life and a desire to communicate, a will to, in spite of her lost language. I'm glad I can alleviate suffering by doing this job for her.

When I return to her flat she's doing her old model's strut for Veta, sashaying along the length of the flat as if it's a runway. Then she does a little dance. She is light on her feet, carrying her weight up high like a bird, dipping and twisting to create flamenco-like movements with her shawl. She's wiry, unstoppable. The railroad flat—long down the middle—is the perfect setting in which to vogue and act sassy.

Issues of placement: these prove the most difficult—more than the language problem; the excess energy in the middle of the night problem; the moments of panic—*Where's the other one* [Gina]? *Who are these people* [the aides]? More than these is this problem of things winding up in the place that seems wrong to me and right to her.

Gina kept saying I didn't get it. The day I moved in I saw that life in Long Island City was utter chaos. There was a profound error in even believing there was anything to be gotten.

Soon I see an intelligence at work. Things are not random or chaotic, necessarily. There is a narrative.

Packing a bag for the park, I ask my mother to put the sketchbook and blanket in the tote. The tote and blanket wind up inside the sketchbook. When I wake up, the cat litter box is missing, or seems so to me. But no, it has been placed on top of the bureau, covered first with a layer of a plastic bag from the deli, then a layer of my shoes, then a layer of her clothing, neatly folded. My shoes keep finding new homes: in the key basket, on my pillow. My pillow winds up on her bed. I come in to the bedroom and both beds have been slept in. The cat, she believes, eats a diet of fruit and milk. I put out cat food and water at night, and in the mornings she replaces it with chopped banana, apple, and milk.

I think of Patañjali's *viparaya*. How many filters of knowing obscure my own experience? What makes my mother's less right than my own? What makes anyone's?

On the street, I hear a woman say to her children, "Move over so that they could get by." The wrong grammar sticks in my head—*wrong to me*. It's not wrong to the woman, who also speaks to her kids in Spanish and then Spanglish. In Spanish, you would say "so that they could get by" and it would be correct, because it's subjunctive. Many things are just a matter of perspective.

I have been exploring options for a place to move my mother when I go back to Penn State for fall semester, in two months, and this seems to have exacerbated her confusions of placement. I show her pictures of my place in State College, and now she thinks we already live there. This seems to make her happy. Perhaps the fantasy is as good as the real thing. If this is delusion—a form of *vikalpa*, perhaps—is it not also serving a purpose?

On a walk out on Vernon she says, "Do you remember, we used to live here." It's as if all minutes exist in one moment.

"You know me, right?" she also asks.

"Yes. And you know me?"

"Yes. But I don't know how I'm going to get where I'm supposed to be." She says, also, "Wow—look at that! Look," but then comes back to this problem of not knowing, and how scary this is: "I used to be here, but I'm not anymore. I'd like to stay with you but I don't know where I'm supposed to go here."

"I'll take care of you."

"Thank you, honey, thank you very much." Then, approaching the apartment's outer vestibule, she tells me, "No, honey, we don't live here anymore, we moved."

There is a desperate panic to her angst. Her lostness has method, if to the unlost person it would be impossible to discern what that method is.

I think what's going on is that she's very upset about Gina's absence. "People could have told me!"

"We did." I have told her that Gina went on vacation, but I fear that the image of Gina as a corpse has had a subliminal effect on my mother and she now believes on some level that she witnessed Gina's death.

"I don't understand." She purses her lips into the shape of a spit, like *This smells bad*, as if the not understanding is a mean trick on her.

※ ※ ※

Perhaps my mother's Alzheimer's-induced psychic despair is only an exaggerated expression of normal human angst. Is there a cure for existential grief? Slow down long enough to think about our deepest fears and there lies the human condition. Aren't we all lost, alone, unconvinced of our true purpose? There is no clear path to relief. Where should we be? Where should we be going? Does any of us know, really?

I've been lost. One time I went for a walk at a wooded writer's colony and couldn't find my way back. I listened for the sound of traffic on a far-away country road, but when I located the source it was actually a stream. My path spiraled. I identified landmarks that looked vaguely but not exactly like ones I'd noticed minutes earlier. Even then—five years ago, two years before the diagnosis—I flashed to an image of my mother lost. She was always getting lost. I'd watched her solve her problems by trusting in fate and following an intuitive course. Fate and intuition were closely related in our family.

Lost in the woods, then, I did the same. And I did find my way. My panic dissipated. My mother used to have this kind of trust in the universe, and so did I. But now I know it's possible to be irrevocably lost, untethered from divine protection and mystical intelligence. Everything has let my family down, even reason.

I practice yoga because at some level I am seeking yoga's essential goal: an experience of the present uncluttered by past or future. This is Samadhi, an enlightened and ecstatic state. That Samadhi is removed from reason and coherence is not, in the yoga texts, regarded as a hindrance. Now I must reconsider everything I thought I believed.

My mother's experience is one of disconnected, separate moments. Even up until a month ago I understood this in a positive light. This is what I wrote about in a piece in the *New York Times* two years ago, "Living in the Moment":

> "*Yoga citta vritti nirodha*—yoga is the cessation of the fluctuations of consciousness. This, from Patañjali's Yoga Sutras, was the first piece of a classical text I memorized when I trained to become a yoga teacher. Perhaps paradoxically, this also seemed to describe what had been happening to my mother.... Now I sometimes believe I am not so much losing my mother as communicating, more and more so exclusively, with that side of her that exists only in the present....To exist outside of memory is to occupy the moment wholly."

Things look different today. The relentless and unforgiving present is a source of panic and terror. That moment is corrupted if it is a moment in perpetual pain.

In class one day, Cyndi says, "seek *nirodha*." She translates this word variously as quiet, space, ease, lack of striving. I think of it as emptiness. Also, I think of it as *cessation*, from that same sutra: Yoga is the cessation of the fluctuations of consciousness. This is B.K.S. Iyengar's translation. There is also: "Yoga is the restriction of the fluctuations of consciousness" (Georg Feuerstein); "Union, spiritual consciousness, is gained through control of the versatile psychic nature" (Charles Johnston); "The restraint of the modifications of the mind-stuff is Yoga" (Swami Satchidananda).

Each time Cyndi refers to quiet and ease I think, grimly, *cessa-*

tion, restriction, control, restraint. I think of a present that contains neither future nor past—a moment so short as to be discontinuous with anything that came before or will come after. It makes me claustrophobic, this present—too fleeting to leave room for an identity of any kind. It is consciousness severed from context.

Three weeks later, Gina comes back from Bellevue saying she wants to stay. It occurs to me that I need a vacation, so I make a plan. I will leave my mother in Gina's care in Long Island City and attend a three-day yoga workshop upstate, out of cell phone range. I build in an extra three days before the workshop on my own at the retreat center. I know this is very irresponsible of me. I seek survival.

It's a bucolic property in Delaware County, New York, with a private guesthouse run by a yoga teacher I know. "No clocks, no TV, no schedule," reads her website. I arrange the day care and home care for the week and beg Gina to troubleshoot on her own if there's an emergency. I will borrow a friend's truck Tuesday and cart in groceries and do yoga and read until the teacher and students arrive Friday. My plan is to drive back to the city Sunday.

Midnight the second night, there is a refreshing summer breeze pushing the curtains into the room, and I am reading from a book of Buddhist proverbs that someone has left behind in my guest room:

> *"It seems that often when problems arise, our outlook becomes narrow."*
> —THE FOURTEENTH DALAI LAMA

"Instead of allowing ourselves to be led and trapped by our feelings, we should let them disappear as soon as they form, like letters drawn on water with a finger."

—DILGO KHYENTSE RINPOCHE

"[R]esourcefulness [means] that you can deal with whatever is available around you and not feel poverty stricken."

—CHÖGYAM TRUNGPA

The present moment need not bring me terror, nor should any future moment. *Stay calm.*

The same wind propels the slightest wisp of a radio signal to my phone, and two startling messages appear. Of course, they are not surprising. I have no right to be taken off guard. One is a text from Gina:

"Mm has disappeared. We were2 go2 fr appt and I left her fast asleep while I ran out. I hid all her shoes."

And there is a phone message from an emergency room doctor at Elmhurst Hospital in Queens: "I'm calling regarding Michele McKee, who has come back to our facility after running into the street at some point today."

My world cracks into many pieces.

It's a mile to the nearest cell phone reception. The moon is bright and I climb to the hilltop without a flashlight. I reach the ER doctor. To him, I was just a phone number. He doesn't even know my name. He found my number because another ER doctor recognized our mother. When she got lost six months ago, police brought her to Elmhurst to check her vitals. Now, she was back. Combing the records by date, the doctor located her chart. The only contact was my telephone—no name.

A doctor *recognized* her, in an ER in New York City.

The doctor suggests we move her from ER to the hospital intake ward. There, he says, a social worker can get involved and help us locate a safe place for her.

As he and I are speaking, I see what is about to occur in a flash, in the instant before it actually happens. We've been rejected for funded home care four times now. I can't solve this problem. Just like that, this doctor will take control of her care, and suddenly our conversation will take place in an entirely different context from the version I'd felt stuck inside only days ago. I experience a grand sense of lightness and weight shed. On the other side of this conversation, I will have passed a turning point beyond which I can never go back. I am no longer my mother's caretaker, nor is Gina.

He says she shouldn't move back home. I tell him that I agree.

I teach my students to write toward epiphany, and this is that. I am moving through a trial that will irrevocably change me. The world is slowly shifting, taking on a different hue.

I feel guilt, and also I feel triumph. And I feel awe. In her state of cognitive arrest, my mother breezed out her door and removed herself from a situation that was unsafe, unhealthy, and unsustainable. After all my acres of information gathering, and Gina's agonizing attempts to maintain her sanity while staying home with her, my mother simply flew out like a little bird and let the world take her into its embrace. *Just relax*! she used to say to us. *Don't worry*! Maybe she can take care of herself better than we can.

🪷 🪷 🪷

Gina is out in the world ten days exactly before she looks back at her shadow and sees the truth: this world is too rough for her. She sends me mood-swinging texts saying she will readmit herself at Bellevue, and then she does. Everyone's in the hospital now.

Within the week, I have given notice for the lease in Long Island City and found a room in assisted living at the beach for my mother. Gina cannot afford the apartment without our mother, and our mother can't afford it on top of assisted living. The facility is very peaceful, at the southern tip of Brooklyn. We can't afford it long, but long enough to figure out something else.

I go to the hospital to accompany my mother on her move to the beach. I discover her wandering the hall by the nurses' station. She is ghostlike, dressed in pale blue hospital flannels and matching blue socks with white rubber dots on the soles for traction. She livens up when she sees me. She hugs me close: "Oh thank god, thank god! Thank god, you're here. I lost all my money. My shoes. Take me home, honey."

The staff lets me try to reach the doctor from the telephone at the nurses' station, and I stand there several minutes on hold while the EMTs and my mother get prepared to leave. As I wait, I reflect with irony that tomorrow is Gina's birthday. I was born exactly two years and two days after she was. I am on hold five minutes, six. I look at the digital reader as it races through the seconds. The date reads 7/21. Then the timer reaches an identical count of 7:21 seconds. I note this distractedly. Then it hits 7:22—Gina's birthday. Then it hits 7:23, 7:24—my birthday. I stay on hold another minute, two minutes. We're into August, now September. I see the whole year slipping by. What will come of the future?

But it is done. Gina left her cat, Cookie, with a friend before rechecking herself into Bellevue. The apartment needs only to be shut down. I have found a subletter to stay out the remaining weeks of the month, and he'll take residence the afternoon of my birthday. Gina and my mother—they're moved out forever. I don't know where Gina will go when she leaves Bellevue, and neither does she. But it's done, here. On my birthday I will work on closing the apartment, the place my mother lived as she slowly lost her mind.

When I arrive at her flat to do so, first thing, the new air conditioner shorts the power strip. It's the second-hottest July week on record ever; the *Washington Post* is calling this "Humigeddon." As soon as I reset the strip, it snaps off again. I set it once more and it flicks off a third time. At its longest, the A/C runs fifteen minutes before it trips the breaker. I feel despair. I remove the other items off the power cord and this enables the A/C to run for several minutes. Then it blows the circuit breaker in the basement.

The cause of the power overload is obvious: minus the plug that still has my DO NOT TOUCH placard, there are only three outlets in the apartment total, and most everything—TV, radio, lights to three rooms—is connected to this one. There is an elaborate daisy chain of power strips and extension cords tenuously holding together everything. By the time I've disassembled the entire network I've collected ten extraneous extension cords. *Ten*. This is a seven-hundred-square-foot apartment. A disordered mind put it together. Problems got fixed by adding to faulty infrastructures.

Another knot of cables lies between the desk—with the computer—and the file cabinet—with the telephone and answering machine. This is like a tight, knotted-up ball of yarn. Knots and tangles grow in the brain during Alzheimer's—amyloid proteins, neurofibrillary tangles. The cords are like a map to the inside of a sufferer's head.

I thread cords out of tangles and loop plugs out of eyeholes. I think, The beginning of the end is a long time away from the end. I feel despair again. It sits in my gut, a dread feeling. In moments the despair lifts and I feel elation: *I am trapped… I will be free.*

I collect two garbage bags of clothes for the thrift store and three of garbage—mostly food I'd ordered for my mother and Gina, a hundred dollars in frozen pork and spinach. I carry them down and leave the garbage on the curb and the clothing in front of a thrift shop around the corner. Just Things, it's called: that's just right. The material world never mattered much to my mother. Once when I was living in California my mother had a piece of family furniture moved out for me, and the shippers lost—or stole—it. "It's just an object," she said.

Just Things is closed, but they'll find the bags in the morning, as if the stork dropped them.

Only after I head across the river on my bicycle do I remember that the weather forecast is for violent storms. Through three days of the heat wave the city has been storing up pressure. I'm back in the East Village sitting on my roof alone, having wine and looking at the sky and celebrating—or not celebrating—my birthday, when I flash back to the bags of clothing at Just Things. Friends have offered to take me out, but it doesn't feel like a time to revel. Gina is still in Bellevue. My mother is in assisted living at the beach, wondering what she's supposed to be doing and when I'll take her home. They are both homeless.

A dog barks from the apartment across the way—lonely, maybe? Where is the owner? How long has he been left alone? There are abandoned, lost creatures everywhere. Who will care for them? A different dog, higher pitched, communicates with the first one across the air. I hear the stray honk of a taxi and the nearing shush of car wheels rolling eastward along the pavement. I stare at roiling clouds in the sky and feel suddenly content. I am grieving, and yet to grieve is to be alive. The despair has turned to something else, an ethereal calm.

The mist has thickened my hair, and my skin feels moist. When the humidity hits 99 percent like this, I feel full and lush. There are the lights of the bridge. I want to eat this moment. My mother loves me. Did I ever doubt it? "It's like a drug," Veta had said, holding old pictures of us. "She talks to you and she calms right down. Pride and joy. Pride and joy."

Then the sky cracks and rain starts sheeting out of it. I think of those garbage bags of clothes at Just Things. Everything has gone to shit. Or maybe this is a cleansing. *Wash the rags in the cool water… Let it run down…* Didn't someone write this into song one time?

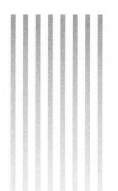

PART THREE
SWEAT

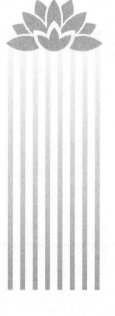

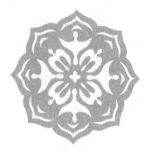

Claire Dederer

The, Um,
Sexy Yoga Essay

When I started doing yoga my husband was very excited. When I say "excited," I don't mean he was happy for me to be getting some healthful exercise, though he was, or that he was enthusiastic about my burgeoning exploration of meditation practice, though he felt pretty OK about that too. No, I mean he was *excited* excited.

After I'd been to five or six classes, we were lying in bed reading one night when he asked, "Um, so what do you do when you're at yoga?" I perked right up. When you start doing yoga you're basically going through your days hoping someone, anyone, will ask you about your practice. It's like having a new boyfriend; you yearn to utter the beloved's name. Also, you can *do* stuff. New stuff. It would be nice to have someone ask about it—let's be honest, it would be nice to brag a bit.

I sat up in bed. "Well!" I said, in the voice of one about to unspool a long recitation. "When we get to class, we unroll our mats and then we sit in meditation for a few minutes. It was really hard for me at first, but now I think I'm really starting—"

He broke in, nicely. "No, I mean, what poses do you do?"

"Well, we do Downward Dog a lot, that's really the basic pose, and we do Bridge, and I tried Eagle and Camel this week." I was warming to my subject and began describing the poses.

"Maybe you could...show them to me?"

"Sure, I'll get my mat out tomorrow."

"No, I mean right now."

Oh. Oh! The penny dropped. And, reader, I did it: I hopped out of bed and—there on the bedroom floor in my shortie pajamas—I did the poses. I did Downward Dog and Upward Dog and Plank and a couple of Warriors and Camel, the porniest pose of all. I would've done Wheel but I couldn't yet manage it. I did them, and my husband watched very, very closely and was very, very happy.

Yoga is sexy. It's an undeniable truth—and one apparently well known to the male population at large—but it's a truth that rarely gets talked about in the yoga world. I've been doing yoga for fifteen years; hell, I wrote a book about yoga. Which is to say, I'm around yoga people a lot. I talk about yoga a lot. I hear about yoga a lot. And I've never heard a single yoga teacher or student acknowledge that yoga is, well, hot. But it is. Very. Need I explain why? For starters, all that arching and twisting and bending. Spread your sitting bones! says the teacher. Open your chest toward the sky! Really, sometimes it feels like all the yoga studio is lacking is a pole and a two-drink minimum. These days, I do hot yoga, so everyone's half-naked and filmed with sweat. Add to that the simple truth that most people simply look better the more yoga they do—backs are straighter, stomachs flatter—and you have yourself a situation. A hotness situation.

And yet. No one at my local studio ever made reference to this hotness. It seemed odd that everyone was pretending yoga was as asexual as Mormon underpants. I for one was a little embarrassed; sometimes spreading my legs and leading with my chest and flipping my hipbones made me feel a little skanky, like one of those bikini-clad chicks at a Hotte Latte stand. But slowly it all began to make sense: if you started worrying about the almost cheesy sexiness of yoga, you'd be too embarrassed ever to do any yoga poses at all.

⁂ ⁂ ⁂

After a while I noticed that there were a couple of ways in which the sexuality of yoga outed itself. I became aware of the first after I'd been doing yoga for a couple of years. I'd heard of some famous teachers and I wanted to watch them teach, and so I hied myself to YouTube. And invariably when I went online—to watch Richard Freeman float through Surya Namaskara A, or to take a virtual class from Kira Ryder, or to listen to what Erich Schiffman had to say about Krishnamurti—the right-hand side of my screen would be filled with thumbnails for, well, smut: Hot Sexy Yoga; Erotic Yoga; Yoga Babes Gone Wild.

It freaked me out a little. Here I was, thinking about my *spiritual practice*, for chrissake, and all of a sudden I found myself confronted with some profoundly waxed, inhumanly sheeny creature doing Dhanurasana in a white G-string. The computer screen, divided between the yoga I came for and the yoga I found, was like a map of the terrible dichotomy of humanity. Our highest selves and lowest selves, side by side, with a Zillow banner ad uniting the two.

The public fascination with the sexual component of yoga also found its expression, I soon discovered, in the recurring narrative of the guru scandal. The guru scandal is always the same, a ritual-ized carnival of humiliation, unspooling in a predetermined sequence of events: some male yoga teacher ascends to the top of his field; it's revealed that he's been getting it on with/sexually harassing his female students; the yoga community expresses dismay and horror; the *New York Times* does a sanctimonious Style section piece on it; that's the last we hear of it, until the next time it happens.

Scandals and pornography: these are the ways sexuality outs itself in a repressed culture—in a religious culture. And yoga is of course a religion, whether or not we choose to partake. Like every other religious community, it has never quite figured out how to deal with sex. It's a little more confusing with yoga because most other religious communities don't *look* quite so sexy. Other religions don't have this particular kind of problem: a firestorm of pervy sports radio jokes when it turns out Lululemon pants are see-through.

And to complicate matters, yoga has a long tradition of being tied to actual sex acts. That tradition is called tantra and I know more about it than I ever want to because: Sting. Most of us aren't interested in tantra and its many, many esoteric practices, including, just as a for-instance, the retention of kundalini energy through nonejaculation. But you don't need to be doing tantra for yoga to seem more sexualized—*much* more sexualized—than other spiritual practices.

When I talk about yoga being sexy, I mean that it looks sexy. But yoga, of course, is not about how stuff looks. It's about how stuff feels. That's what we keep returning to, over and over in our yoga practices: we try to get at how things feel. And I wonder if there's a kind of sexual feeling to yoga.

Here's why I wonder: because studios are filled with thirty- and forty-something women who seem to be, well, in love with yoga. Who treat it like their secret boyfriend or girlfriend. Who plot and scheme and hire help to get out of the house to get to yoga. When they talk about yoga, their eyes shine. They use words like *delicious* and *addiction*. They buy new outfits. They feel seen, as one does with a new love, even if the eyes seeing them are their own, in the studio mirror. Do these women have all these same feelings about their longtime husbands or partners? I will go out on a limb and say: they do not! These women are besotted, which is not exactly how marriage works.

Flaubert famously said, "Madame Bovary, c'est moi" and these yoga ladies, compulsively drawn to the sensations they discover and explore on the mat, well, c'est moi. I am one of them. Have been one of them. Will be one of them. And there's something we're all finding in yoga class. It's not sex, exactly. But it might be sex's kissing cousin.

This was made abundantly clear to me recently when I found myself attempting Visvamitrasana. Every Monday night I take a break from my usual hot yoga vinyasa studio to attend my local gym, where an advanced class is taught by a quiet, slightly simian-looking genius by the name of Jorge. Jorge likes to organize his classes around a single pose. He'll spend weeks and weeks working toward something tough, preparing you, easing you into it. A kind of seduction.

Toward the end of class one day Jorge led us into Visvamitrasana, in which you lunge, tuck your shoulder under your leading leg, balance on that forward arm and your aft leg, and grab your leading foot with your upper hand. You lift your foot from the ground with your hand, and then twist the whole contraption toward the sky, pulling your torso through the arc made by your upper arm and leg. Really, save us both a lot of trouble and just go look it up.

If it sounds like a difficult posture, it's even worse than it sounds. As we pulled into the pose, Jorge said gently, almost inaudibly, "What does it feeel like? What are you feeeling?" Jorge always asks this question, with the "e" drawn out in a manner that's, well, feelingful. The whole point, says Jorge, is to feeel something.

And Jorge is right. I mean, this is what yoga is supposed to do in general. It says so right there in Sutra 1.2: "Yoga is to still the patterning of consciousness." (This from the lovely and essential translation by Chip Harntraft.) In other words, we do yoga in order to move past the mind's perceptions into actual experience.

Visvamitrasana is a stern teacher when it comes to Sutra 1.2. There's no way to escape feeling when you're doing it; as for the patterning of consciousness, you can't even remember that the freaking patterning of consciousness even *exists* because you no longer have any idea which foot is which, or which hand is which. This time I was ready to assume the pose, thanks to Jorge's prep, and I balanced there for long, sweet moments, exposed as anything, tangled in my own limbs. It wasn't an arousing experience, but it wasn't *un*arousing. I suppose it was, lord help me, sensual.

God, what a terrible, terrible word. *Sensual.* It makes a person think of creepy dudes offering massages, and of ladies in caftans seducing pool boys, and of marriage manuals instructing wives to wrap themselves in cellophane. Or maybe that's just me. There's something skeezy about that word, but it's just plain true: yoga is sensual. Voluptuous. Embodied. We all have a deep need to be in our bodies, experiencing them with immediacy. Unhindered by the patterning of consciousness. Sex does that for us; so does yoga. So do all kinds of other things, from skiing to knitting; sex and yoga just both happen to be incredibly efficient at it. I felt that as I lifted into Visvamitrasana: total presence; total immediacy.

More than a decade has gone by since that first night when my husband asked me to do the poses for him. Now he goes to yoga with me. He huffs and sweats and twists and arches and, yes, spreads his sitting-bones. I don't fool myself that he's immune to the hotness on display in that room; he has, after all, confessed to a crush on our teacher Jen. (Every right-thinking human has a crush on our teacher Jen.) But as he makes his way through the poses, one after another, he's pretty busy just trying to do the yoga. Like all of us, he's just trying to feel something.

Brenda Miller

Everyday Yoga: Three Poses

Canine Yoga

My dog Abbe arrived in my home on January 3, 2007. Almost four months old, a seven-pound bundle of energy and curiosity, she didn't understand me too well, and I didn't understand her. She couldn't comprehend collars and leashes and commands to sit. Neither could I. She felt it appropriate to pee in the kitchen and to gnaw contently on a doorframe. I felt these behaviors were completely inappropriate, but didn't know how to get the point across in her language. We walked in the park while it snowed, and her paws iced over.

We made a lot of mistakes. We each thought the other was kind of goofy, so we accepted the mistakes with good humor. We didn't hold them against each other.

She got sleepy a lot. She could go from full tilt to full-on snoring in less than a minute.

Now, we understand each other much better. For instance, for New Year's weekend, I traveled with Abbe to Port Townsend, stayed in a little apartment by the bay. When we arrived, Abbe clearly asked me for something. And I understood, after a few daft minutes, what it was she wanted. I then fulfilled her need—it was a simple one, after all—and then we took a nap.

We had traveled from Bellingham, by car and by ferry, bought groceries at the coop, and Abbe had waited (not so patiently) all that time to get out of the car. I brought in our things while Abbe sniffed out the place, then immediately headed to bed. I put the lavender eye pillow on my face, tried to settle into a resting pose, but Abbe whined—a distinct, urgent whine—from the kitchen.

I got up. She got up and stared at me intently. I moved toward the sink and Abbe moved with me, hurried around to plant herself squarely in front of me, whined again. Of course: water. I filled her water bowl, set it down, and she lapped it all up, gulping as if she were dying of thirst. Back to bed: now we could all relax. She settled herself against my legs, let out a sigh. No reproach. Just happiness that she'd eventually gotten what she needed. No more, no less.

I would like to be so accepting. I've found often I don't really know what I need and so become vaguely dissatisfied with everything I receive. I mutter in my head a list of grievances. Whining, but not the clear, unambiguous whine of my dog. No, this whine is petulant, childish. And if I do finally receive what I think I need, it is tainted with this aura of complaint.

I'd like to let Abbe be my yoga teacher, to help me recognize when I'm whining and how to turn that whine into something clearer, more conducive to exchanges of truth: no grudges, no grievance. In yoga I'm learning to listen to the truth of my body, but also to what my heart so clearly communicates. It can be so nuanced, this listening: you need to grow very quiet and concentrate at that edge between striving and acceptance, the boundary line between productive and unproductive pain.

The other day, as I tried to push myself up from full belly into a hovering Plank, I involuntarily let out a loud "ooof" as I found myself stuck on the ground. I started laughing, my neighbor started laughing, and soon the entire class was laughing at this simple truth, this acceptance: the pose is hard. All we can do is try.

Yin Yoga

I feel like I worked harder these past few months than I've ever worked before. Nothing extraordinary, really, but the stuff of a full life, a life that remains interesting by constantly challenging me.

Yesterday I took a breath. And in that breath, I felt vulnerability flood through my body. An ache that makes your heart tweak. An openness that scares you. A trembling in your upper arms. A twinge behind your eyes.

This is what happens in yin yoga. In yin yoga, you hold a pose for a long time, maybe five minutes, maybe ten. You breathe deep and settle in. You find your edge. You surrender and let the body do its own yoga for a while. The connective tissue stretches. The body unwinds, unravels. Your teacher tells you stories to keep your mind out of it.

And then you slowly come out of the pose. Your limbs remember they are part of you. And a vulnerable ache will often bloom there, right where you opened up.

It passes. You go on to the next pose. But you remember it, deep in your cells. You remember the space that exists there, below the level of bone and flesh. It beguiles and scares you at the same time.

This is the consequence of opening.

My work often feels like this. As if I've been holding a pose for a long time, pressing myself to the edge without quite being aware of it. It's only when I stop that I realize how deep I've gone. And when I come back to myself, it can be a little disconcerting, as if I don't recognize this self that has returned.

I have to be gentle. Move slowly. Resist the urge to create work in order to avoid this vulnerable space. Just breathe. Look up. Go out on the deck. Walk the dog in this air that is bright, but still cold. Notice. Simply notice that I am back in the world, and say, "Welcome."

Accidental Yoga

Last week, I accidentally took a power yoga class.

Now understand: I have always emphatically said I am *not* a "power yoga person." I had a pretty clear idea of power yoga people: tattooed, lithe, ultraserious, and out of their minds.

I arrived at the yoga studio early, pleased that I had made it to the 5:30 "intuitive flow" class with my favorite teacher, Amy. (I hadn't felt well all day, and it would have been easy enough to stay home.) And there was Amy at the front desk, checking people in, with her calm smile, her effusive greeting. I signed in, and bustled into the studio...

...where a blast of hot air greeted me. Where a harmonium sat at the front of the room. Where all the mats were lined up in an unfamiliar pattern.

I went back out front. "Amy, am I in the right class?"

"Power yoga?" she answered cheerfully.

"No, I wanted to be in *your* class."

"I don't teach until 7:15."

At which point my brain got all twisted up. My brain wanted to argue with Amy, to tell her she had it wrong, that she had to teach at 5:30 because, after all, *I was here for her 5:30 class.* My brain clicked back through the schedule and realized I was a few days off: that Amy's 5:30 class is always on *Tuesday,* not Thursday. But my brain knew that my desire for a 5:30 class on Thursday had blocked my knowledge that no 5:30 class existed.

And that's when fear kicked in. That's when the brain went into heavy whining mode: *I can't do power yoga. It's too hot. I'll throw up. I'll make a fool of myself. I don't want to do power yoga. Don't make me do power yoga!*

Amy looked up from the computer. "Don't worry," she said, "You can totally do it." Then she flashed me that smile. Who can argue with that smile?

So I slunk back into the studio, set my mat in the far back corner, and waited for my torture to begin. I looked around, and sure, there were some lithe tattooed people, but there were also a lot of people who looked just like me.

The teacher, Paul, started us slowly. He read Rumi to us. Something about love and wine and letting go (very Rumi). He had a beautiful voice. I began to trust a little, and then a little more. He said

Yoga, no matter what style, is always about meeting yourself where you are. Hello self, I said, here we are.

And yes, there we were, together, my cranky self and I, flowing through one Sun Salutation, then another, the heat rising through every part of me, sweat beading then flowing down my back; there we were breathing deep and bowing into Child's Pose for a quick rest before joining the others, then flowing easily into Camel Pose and back into Child.

At the end he played that harmonium and I understood harmony. I heard my own voice resonating there with the others. And I was glowing: with sweat, yes, but also with the joy that comes from doing something you never thought you could do. The accidental, the unexpected, the parting of your own stolid ways.

When I went out to the lobby to put on my shoes, I told Amy I loved it. And with her same calm smile she said, "There must have been some reason you got confused this week."

So, here's to confusion. Here's to the accidental. Here's to finding out what happens when the universe changes your plans.

Alan Shaw

Broga

I like yoga in the way most culture-slumming smart people say they like watching pro wrestling: I enjoy the physical experience of it and I don't care about the message. I know my attitude is wrong. I know I'm missing out on something important here. I know most of my yoga peers sneer at me for being a tourist, and not in it for the *namaste*, but I can't get past my premise. Let me explain.

I started practicing yoga a few years ago after suffering a humiliating but crippling back injury. I had gone home to see my parents for Thanksgiving, and spent most of the visit playing with one of my nieces. She was a baby at the time. Chubby she was, but baby chubby. I think it was during a spirited game of upsy-daisy that I bent to pick her up, and while trying to stand and upsy-daisy her, I felt something give out.

No, *giving out* is too gentle a description of what my back did. I felt the parliament of ligaments and muscles in my lower back pass an emergency vote to return me to the floor to better think about my life, and then I felt those muscles begin smashing my spine with hammers. It was humbling to learn that I'd disregarded the state of my back for so long and so criminally that I could wreck it while trying to lift my toddler niece.

After much whining and a week in a back brace, I decided to give yoga a try. At the time I was working weekends at The Dragon's Tale, a comic book shop in Neptune Beach, Florida. Two doors down from our shop was a studio called Bikram Yoga Jacksonville. Before my first class, I didn't know anything about Bikram Choudhury and his litigious practices, multimillionaire status, or celebrity courting. I didn't know what some in the American yoga community think of him: that his crassness, his copyrighting yoga postures, and his Rolls Royce collection are decidedly unyogic.

All I knew about the studio is that Rob, the owner, never gave me a hard time about my cigarette butts outside his studio, always had something nice to say to me, and invited me to class at least once a week. He even kept from snorting when I said I'd tried yoga once with Nintendo's Wii Fit. So, my aching lower back in hand, I slid on some gym shorts and tried my first class.

This introduction to yoga, the style and its distinctly physical impact on my body, may explain why my understanding of yoga has remained so firmly rooted in the body. Bikram yoga, with its 105-degree studios and equally severe humidity levels, molds the body first and spirit far later. I think that you can't not appreciate yoga on a physical level when your body is otter-slick and lobstered from the heat.

I can't see or feel my spirit wiggling to stay in Toe Stand, but I can feel my body trying to. I don't have any sense of inner peace, of centeredness, or mindfulness when I flex and twist into Full Cobra, but I know what my back is doing. It's envying the plastic-spined cheerleader three mats down my row who can lift her entire chest off the floor. The show-off.

I also like to think that your first yoga session is a lot like your first time watching *Doctor Who*. That first style, much like your first Doctor, is the one you imprint on and the one against which all future styles and Doctors are measured. Mine were Bikram and David Tennant, so I can't help but compare all others to them and observe how not like Bikram or Tennant they are.

☙ ☙ ☙

It's because of this preoccupation with the body that I wonder if yoga would be better off, when trying to attract men, if it were repackaged. Just a skosh.

Call it Broga. Just a bunch of dudes and their mats, stretching and twisting to killer abs and stronger, more limber backs. We could even listen to "Reign in Blood" by Slayer or other melodic speed metal tracks.

Seriously, this could work. Metal chords lead to metal backs, bros!

We start with breathing exercises, but change them to rhythmic headbanging. Breathe in for ten, then headbang out that breath for ten.

The Downward Facing Dog could be retitled Hellhound Faces Home.

Back Bends, call them Arch Enemy.

Happy Baby? Hell, no! Lamb of God!

Tree Stand? No, Murdertree Stand.

Deadman Pose? Damn right, Deadman Pose. Or Cannibal Corpse.

This opinion about yoga does cause some conflict in my life, mostly with my girlfriend. Me, I'm all about the physical. The Broga. I never look for my center and I prefer shoe gazing to navel, unless I'm trying to find out how large my muffin top is today.

For my girlfriend, Dru, her reasons for practicing are all about yoga's ability to center her mind and return her to a peaceful state. A once-weekly, ninety-minute session realigns her spiritual ballast, leaving her stable and mindful for the week ahead. It's a bleed valve for all the chaotic and distracting waste that modern life accumulates in all of us.

We've talked about this during our time together. I start whining about my back or ribs aching, and she says go to yoga.

She tells me about how it will help with my anxiety and hyper-activity, but all I can say back is that it will tighten my core.

I know in those moments she's struggling to think of all the reasons she's still with me, why she still loves me: an emotional kludge debasing the thing that tethers her to her spirit.

Likely, she's a better person than me. But what's more likely is that she knows I have the potential, like all people, to relax, to let the Om begin, to get out a spiritual shovel and dig deeper. To allow the shell that I call home to blossom open and let something touch me.

And to be more honest, I envy her openness to yoga. Her ability to be so emotionally laid bare. I think it's similar to how easily she's touched by anything emotional.

She cries at all the sad parts in movies. She cries at all the uplifting and inspirational moments, too. However crude or seemingly insignificant. Show her a video of a puppy trying to climb up a shallow stair and her eyes start bubbling up tears, even before she can shout, "Honey, I'm not crying."

I never get the vapors from stuff like this; well, almost never. The first ten minutes of *Up* certainly hit me, but only the disturbed and the dumb can get through that prologue with dry eyes.

But what's more, I think that some of us will always struggle with feeling their emotions the way she can. It seems that some of us are born with a deeper emotional register, like me. That's not to say that we can feel with more sophistication, but that we need more to make us feel something.

Something like what yoga brings into our lives.

People like Dru, they get it from the first breathing pose and the last floor-rocking asana. They ride their emotions like a stallion, while everyone else, me included, we have to coax that filly out.

Not long after we started dating, I got a sense of Dru's reverence for yoga, what the cause of it might be: I found a picture of her while Facebook-stalking her. (And don't get all rubbery over that phrase; Facebook is the modern equivalent of surreptitiously asking a friend about the girl at the end of the bar. Facebook handles the sneaky questions about the social history of a prospective date. And we say far more about ourselves on Facebook than we realize, or at least our pictures do.)

I knew I already liked the girl after our first date at her house, when she cooked three delicious courses with all the effort of Julia Child scrambling eggs late one Sunday morning. I'm such a sucker for a home-cooked meal, it's a wonder I haven't dropped to bended knee for the Food Network. And I would marry Alton Brown in a second, damn what the world and his wife think of our love. It's pure!

But the night Dru hooked me by the heart grew long, words and kisses were exchanged; then she tossed me out. She had an anatomy test in the morning and all of my cheap lines no longer worked. The inevitable Facebook friending followed, and that was how I found her yoga pictures album.

She has half a hundred photos from her more active yoga days. Most were taken in late 2005, when she'd returned from a semester abroad. While studying in Prague she reconnected with yoga after flirting with it all through her late teens and early twenties. The classes were taught in a quaint but humble studio, and each cost about two dollars American.

Dru had been injured in a car accident in her teens, and from that point on required almost weekly chiropractic adjustments. She'd not been able to get them as easily in Prague, and so she walked into that yoga studio. By the time she finished her undergrad studies a year later, she was teaching yoga classes weekly. The pictures were taken from those days.

One picture slayed me. Dru is in a south Tampa yoga studio, a few years younger than she is now, her hair noticeably shorter. The picture shows her hovering over the floor. Wearing a red top and pink yoga pants, she's inclined forward in Eight-Angle Pose. She holds her upper body in a lowered push-up position, and has her legs bent around to her right. One leg is fed under her arm and the other over, and she's twisted them at the ankle.

I've seen her in this pose in three other photos from the album, and each one just knocks me out. The casual strength it must have taken, the years of focusing on her core, her form. She's exhibiting in the photos the strength I chase each time I practice yoga. The power in her body I see each time I look at this photo kills me and reminds me of why I fell for her.

It's in her eyes. She's looking at the camera, face placid as a still lake at dawn. No sweat on her brow, or grimace marring her mouth, no red flushing across her cheeks.

She's at peace.

And there's no pride in her expression.

I want to think that most people who can strike these power poses wear an expression, intentionally or not, that begs the world to take notice, that says, *Look at this, man. Can you do this? Didn't think so.*

The callous pride I saw in some of the pictures on Bikram Choudhury's website, and in countless other yoga photos I've seen, is not in evidence in Dru's pictures. There's joy in her eyes that she achieved something worth doing because it's so damn hard. But even that conjecture feels off, like I've missed something.

I think what I see in her eyes is an invitation. *Anyone can do this*, she seems to be saying, and she's proving it. Hers is an egoless and serene confidence that is infectious, even to a cynic like me.

Jason Tucker

Bodies of Work: A Mandala

Posture of the Devoted

Assume any position. Persist in it until it feels like you can't do it anymore. Keep doing it until it feels like you can do it again. On the other side of the pain, glimpse something that glitters and looks like the secret to everything. This could be anything. It really doesn't matter what. Even if you don't choose something, something will present itself. If you aren't careful, you may end up choosing something imaginary, or you may lend imaginary significance to some meaningless thing. You may even end up choosing the pain itself. Believe in it. Pursue it as if it were the only desirable destination. Know that soon, like the others you've seen, you will begin becoming the kind of person who pursues that thing. Contort your body and mind into whatever shapes best serve that thing. Find others whose vision is as narrow and distant as your own. Join them in praising one another. Do not acknowledge that such praise of others is really only praise of yourself. Further praise yourself for recognizing a distant light the ignorant are unable to see. Begin to pity them.

I've watched my parents settle into rhythms that seem alternately sustaining and stagnating. Early on, it seemed decided that my ways would depart from their ways. I still watch my father's body, strengthened by his work, yet worn down like a grinding wheel from the same work that carved him. I watch my mother grow ever wearier of her work, yet she remains faithful to it. She keeps the liquor store shelves stocked and immaculately dusted, crafts her own posterboard signs for what the Alabama ABC says is on special, shoos away the alley drinkers when they've had a half-pint too many or when they try to hustle for change in the parking lot. She pities them, and anyone else who doesn't work well or enough or at all. She feels the same about anyone who can't manage drugs or alcohol or money or a marriage or a respectable degree of housework—all the things she has firmly under control, either by abstention (the first two, except for the very occasional drink) or by her constant labors (everything else). Her favorite adjective is *pitiful*. She's been dutifully biding most of her life this way, waiting for the work to be over, waiting for my father's to be over, waiting on him to feel ready to leave their homestead of thirty years. Sometimes she's like a bottle much too big for what's kept in it—fretful over all it has not yet been given to contain.

It wasn't the work itself that drove them, exactly, though they were proud of their accomplishments. Daddy's thing was self-sufficiency. They raised our little homestead out of the hostile Alabama woods pretty much by themselves. Mama really didn't want to move forty miles away from her family to live in a different kind of lonely, beautiful, unwelcoming place. For her mostly-coal-mining family, work wasn't self-reliance; it was sacrifice. It's what you did because you had to do it. It's what good people did. Life was whatever fit in around its edges. Work took whatever time it wanted, and you kept what was left. Work and life were separate things, and it was always sinful to shirk your work. Work won't wait. Unless you're dead or dying, life generally will. She's still waiting to retire so her life can begin. Without sacrifice, my mother wouldn't know what to do with herself.

Since Alabama's state government has a monopoly on liquor sales, her job was a state job with state benefits, one of which matched her contributions to a college fund for me. Thanks to that, and only that, I became the only person in my family (apart from one cousin-nurse) to go to college. She toiled to save the money and to keep the job that offered the benefit. And I am grateful. When I was born, she told my father, "This child's going to make a living with his brain." She's recounted that many times since.

Posture of the Watchful Child

Reach upward, because everything and everyone of importance is bigger than you. Observe the virtuous toils of your people. Feel your father's hand like a leather work glove filled with rebar and unshelled hickory nuts. Notice how the body-shop chemicals have opened cracks, and how the paint and grime settles into them, staining them permanently. His hands will only be clean when he sheds the last of those layers of skin. Examine the functional engineering of your mother's nails—thicker than most screwdriver blades, arched down the center and curved like the beak of a highly specialized tropical bird. One is dark where a heavy thing she was carrying or opening pried it away from the flesh underneath. On your own hands, examine the absence of things to examine. Regret that they appear unwise and unuseful.

I knew I was messing with some kind of brake. I could hear the parts moving behind the wheels when I stepped on the pedal. But I couldn't figure out why the pedal on the John Deere seemed divided but bridged by a steel tab. "What's that?" I asked Daddy when he was busy with something important about the tractor. He barely broke a stride as he flipped the tab that uncoupled the pedals, revealing separate pedals for separate left and right brake systems. It made steering much easier, I eventually figured out. The man you'd misknow if you only knew him by the skill of his hands didn't look up and only said, as he turned back to his business, "Use your head." He said that a lot.

When I was about thirteen—I don't know what started the conversation—I worked up to the edge of hostile adolescent tears and told Mama that I wanted something better than working on cars for a living. Nobody had ever suggested I work on cars for a living. I used the word *better*. Daddy was right over there in his recliner, and I know he heard me, but I didn't look at him and he didn't look at me and we all went back to watching television and none of us ever talked about it again.

Posture of the Assisted Wrench
Stand at ease but attentive, still too small but now eye level with the hands of your father. He will demonstrate much magic. Really, though, he will demonstrate much physics, geometry, engineering,

ingenuity. He will improvise with whatever scrap is at hand. He will discover his own ways of mixing and applying body filler, paint. He will compensate for humidity, temperature, the accidental contamination of his own sweat. Chemistry. Very early, you will learn leverage from him. He will show you how the box end of one wrench can marry the crescent end of another to either break the stubborn nut or snap the bolt in two. Or inadvertently break the heavy steel bench vise, as he will do occasionally. You notice his secret intimacies with tools and wood and cast-off metal. Those few you are able to decipher, you will expect to carry with you and use until you die. The many more you can't will die when he does. Notice the hermitic dignity of what he has earned. Notice the scant rewards he will get for it. Notice how, during those years he works for other men, the shop's owner will need him more than the other way around. One day, his paychecks will begin to bounce and he will clear back some of the woods to build his own shop in the back yard.

Mama always talked about what Daddy could have done if they'd have moved away from this town. He was an expert paint and body man. He'd mastered conventional techniques and invented his own. He had intricate systems known only to him. How they could have moved up to a suburb around Birmingham—some place with a hospital and without so much solitude—and he could be in charge of people or he could be teaching people, even though he'd have hated both of those things.

Posture of Medicinal Labor
Stand. Get up. Get to moving around. Don't just lay up in the bed, at the house, under the air conditioner. That's why you're feeling so

bad. You must work because you will quickly decline and decay—in mind and body and spirit—without it. In the bed is sloth and sickness and disease. At the house are idleness and uselessness and slow-growing dementia. You've seen this in the homes of the elders and the drunks and the unstable unemployable. Under the air conditioner are the weak and the old or the luxuriating, the spoiled, and the idle. You may have the bed and the house and the air conditioner, but only at the close of the day, after you have gone out and earned them.

Growing up out alone in the woods, I often felt mopey and purposeless. One year we planted corn in the field behind the house. It was a garden, but calling it that might give you the wrong idea about the size. It was about 120 yards long and about 30 yards wide. There was still some dark, Black Belt topsoil left, but after years of planting, it had steadily reverted to the hard red clay underneath. I'd never helped with the gardening before. I might have been eleven. Daddy cut furrows behind the tractor with the disk while me and Mama worked up and down in rows, making little holes, dropping three corn kernels inside, and covering them over again. None of us talked. We just worked. Neither of them could ever stand just doing nothing.

In later months and years of planting, hoeing, and harvesting, the same system of daunting pain and soothing satisfaction was always a part of it. The blisters from the hoe handle, steadily working them bigger because there's a lot more chopping of dirt to be done. The weight of your own body as it bends and crouches to long processions of plants waist-high and lower. All the biting, poisonous things that thrive here despite the pesticides. You forget the pain of the sun as the work goes on. With the work, you forget the back pain and the horseflies and the otherwise constant fear of sunning snakes. But you are intermittently reminded, especially when you get to the end of a row, look down the next empty one, and crumble at how far it looks to the other end, especially when you're working in 10-inch increments. By the time it started to get dark, Daddy was spreading the last of the 13-13-13 fertilizer and the whippoorwills had started. The rhythm of the work had left me in a pleasant stupor, even as I braced my lower back with my hand like old men did. The punishing heat of the day had broken and the sweat was gone and the thick air held on like comfortable clothing as the heat leached out of the new-plowed ground and carried the rich, reassuring, dusty smell to meet the bold song of the nighthawk, who sang alone but never did sound lonesome to me. I started to think warmly toward farm work for a moment, of the rewards of owning your own land and working it yourself, but the mosquitoes turn up to plague intensity at dusk, and that helped bring me out of it. And my open blister was bleeding.

On the walk back to the house, Daddy said, "It'll make your food taste better when you have to work for it."

Posture of the Individually Responsible

Whatever the work, point your face toward it. Look at it. Don't look up from it. Keep your mind on it. Work is to be done because work must get done and you can't expect anybody else to do it for you. You will know your body intimately as you mind your business, and this is good. But if it begins to complain, you must not. Unless you are dead, dying, or dismembered, you must work through it. Regardless of its contortions, your body will eventually submit to your will. Weaknesses of will and body aren't natural; they are cultivated, as are strong ones. Complaints signal weakness. Weakness signals laziness. These are all things any person can control.

Mama's brother got hurt in the mines when a high-pressure hydraulic hose ruptured and the loose end whipped him in the eye. He got to keep the eye, but had to quit work for a while. The foreman said they had to hire two people to do the work he'd been doing. Everyone said with pride what a good worker he was. Nobody said that he should have been getting paid twice as much. Hard work started to look like its own reward, because nobody else was going to give you anything for it.

Hard work was also its own punishment. All my father's life, he'd strived to work for no one but himself. The wasted energies of military life just made no sense to him. Though he made staff sergeant, he remembers it as just moving large dirt piles from one end of the yard to the other and back again. Bosses and employees and peers always let him down. Someone else's incompetence cost him the tip of his little finger on an oil rig in Louisiana. He figured he'd better come on home before the work took more of him. For him, the only work worth doing was for yourself. Eventually, when he built the shop behind the house with his own two hands and an arc welder, he felt like he didn't have a choice. Look at how useless it was working for somebody else.

I liked the look of the wide plane of grass around the house just at dusk after I'd finished cutting it. I liked putting parts together the right way. I liked using the bush axe to clear briars and undergrowth, working out the fury that builds naturally during those terrible middle years of school. Such satisfaction was always fleeting. The grass grew so quickly you could practically hear it. The briars always came back as soon as you turned around. Nobody but you, and maybe your father, could tell or would care how well you put something together. His bodywork was meticulously "better than factory," but nobody else could tell the difference. People loved the candy-glass smoothness of his work, but no one, not even me, could truly appreciate its nuances. They'd wreck it again. Or they wouldn't wash it. Or they'd wash it improperly, or worse, run it through the car wash with its brushes and slapping cloth, which collected dirt from other cars and slapped yours with it, like sandpaper tearing at what you'd labored so long and so cleverly to get smooth.

One brutal August, sunshine sharp as a bush axe blade, Daddy wanted me to carry a five-gallon bucket of lime around the house, scattering handfuls between the cinder block pillars that were our only foundation. I told him no. I reasoned with him. "If you had a choice, would you?" He didn't answer, and ended up just doing it himself. We never talked about it. I never refused him again, but he also never asked me for much. He'd never asked me for anything, really.

I was finishing high school and looking toward college and not deciding on a career. I wanted to let Daddy know how much I respected his work, but I didn't know how to say it. I think I just said something like "You do good work."

He's sharp about context and subtext. Around our silent dinner table, he and I have subtle conversations with our eyes in a language my mother can't seem to speak. He said, "You go out and get yourself a job under an air conditioner." I repeated that to people all throughout college. Sometimes it felt like a burden. I didn't know many people with jobs like that.

Posture of the Stiff-Bristled Push Broom

Start here, in the morning, first thing. The concrete floor is smooth and expansive, but filled with obstacles—the lift, the jack, the grease pit; the hand truck, the loading ramps, the cases of liquor; the forklift, the pallets of inventory, the workers going about their business and their smoking, which continually ruin *your* floor; the other, smaller floors cluttered with the dusty remains of lives people abandoned in self-storage units. Do your work well. No one will notice it and no one will thank you. Those are not reasons to do things. This is the kind of work you always start with—work for the children and the unskilled and the untrustworthy—yet you must never consider yourself above it. Despite your ascension, you must never find shame in getting behind the broom, for the sweeping must be done, and you must never hold yourself above any work that any other must do in your service.

Don't try to sweep only the filth you can see. You must cover the floor as thoroughly as if you were painting it. Beware the shop fans, and the hot winds blowing in from outside. They will undo your work. Use the air currents to your advantage. Be methodical. Work in one direction. Start in a corner. Work along the wall. Feel the weight and balance of this most basic tool. Find your grip. It will be the same each time. Find your angles. They will differ with the consistency of the filth at hand. Learn the rhythm. Stroke by stroke, move from one side to the other. The body will learn, and soon proceed without command. The mind will clear, and be at peace, so long as you do not submit to the seduction of pride and remain unresentful of the status of your task.

Everything had to be clean in the body shop, and entirely

dustless in the paint booth. I got a lot of practice at this one summer. Daddy wouldn't let me work until I was sixteen because he wanted me to have one more year of "being a kid."

I spent the summer working in the shop with him and his crew to save up money for parts for the 1969 Plymouth Barracuda that Mama's daddy had given me as an early inheritance. It already had one of Daddy's paint jobs on it. He helped me pay for a new engine and showed me how to overhaul every part of that car. I drove it to college.

Posture of the Infuriated Grease Monkey

In college, I got a part-time job in an express lube. My hands were a bit more scarred and callused and burned now, but I still knew I'd never get hands like the hands of the people I worked with. And I was glad. They knew it too, and seemed glad for me, even though they'd cuss the presumably ungrateful college kids driving new SUVs on Mama and Daddy's dime. I was a college kid, but the guys in the shop didn't treat me like they treated the college-kid customers. They treated me like one of their own who was getting out.

Scream from the grease pit at some Pontiac engineer you've never met when you lay eyes on another goddamn Sunfire. Scratch your unhealed forearm in memory of the last one. Explain to the new guy that it's from the location of the oil filter, that you have to lay your arm across the woven steel of searing hot flex-pipe exhaust in order to get to it. Engineer must have caught his wife fucking a mechanic. Have whole lists of vehicles categorized by the pain they can cause you. Speak only of these things. Keep silent about the physical strength and endurance you have gained in return for your labors. Squint to cry the hot, burnt oil out of your eyes. Make jokes of simultaneous pride and misery.

One day, the owner fired another guy my own age. "I'm sorry, but we just don't have enough work coming in right now," he said. Then he turned to me: "But I can't fire you; you work too hard."

To be fired is supposed to be a punishment, you say, so we need to change the definition. You don't get to go home when you get fired. Soon it catches on with everybody around the shop: You're fired; you have to work Saturday. Understand that your job at the shop is part time, and that your college is full time. Understand that however greasy and scarred and burned you become, this is temporary and everyone knows it. Accept that the full-timers and long-timers have set you apart from the college kids, who never had to work for anything, who don't even know what real work is. Wonder why your coworkers seem comfortable that you will only share their work for three more years. Think they are treating you like a diplomat, dispatched from their country to represent them in another. Doubt that you are adequately qualified.

Posture of the Confidently Resigned

Observe yourself in mid-motion, whatever that motion is. Feel the comfort of its well-practiced arc. See in it the ways in which your father moves. Begin to gain mastery. Know your body well by now, and know the extent to which you can and can't control it. Where before was only force and desire is force when necessary, cut by nuance, subtlety, finesse. Know much better now just how far you have not yet gone. Notice what happens in time away from your discipline—how quickly your proficiency declines. Realize it is only the continued work that allows you to continue the work. Begin work that is not the work of the hands or the back or the sweat glands. Identify patterns that run beneath all the labors you've done and seen. Know, despite this, that you will be unable to sustain them all equally. You must choose. Alter your definitions of work and of air conditioners. Remain unwilling to define this new work as more valuable than—or even equal to—that of your people, even if some of them tell you otherwise. Even if you once told your father otherwise. Forever regret that.

Posture of the Dutiful Human Being
Nod in acknowledgment to other workers. Don't necessarily smile. Scowl toward the shirkers. We ain't got much use for anybody who wants to lay out of work. Your body and your mind and your people will punish you for it. Work must be done because it is immoral to avoid it. Others suffer their own labors, and as you are no better than they, it is your duty to labor among them. Otherwise you only add to their burdens, become a parasite on their tithes and their taxes, an ungrateful living insult to their discipline and dependability. And so when you encounter another at their labor, whatever their labor, offer a solemn and knowing and respectful expression. Give a subtle, manly wave to the road crew. Apologize when you need to interrupt anyone working behind a counter or a desk. Do not make the lives of good service people—or any other good worker—more difficult than they have to be. Make your respectful displays clear but brief. Workers at work are not to be disturbed beyond the briefest of unspoken acknowledgments. But the opposite is also true. Bad workers, bad service, bad attitudes must be punished boldly, bitterly, resentfully. In the manner and degree of punishment, use your own discretion.

All my male cousins are working men. Erek comes from Mama's side, and works at a factory that makes valves and valve controls that direct fluids through everything from sewers and coal mines to gas stations and beverage systems. He wrote about his work in his Facebook statuses several months after his father, my uncle, died at the end of a decade-long argument with leukemia. I cleaned up his punctuation and such. He'd appreciate that.

Nov. 20, 2012: Hey, it's me again!!!! Just wanted to let everybody know it was a long hard fun day of work. I wish it was longer. If I could, I would work six days a week and 23 and a half hours a day. The other half that makes up the whole 24 is for peeing and #2. There is no time for nothing else. Not even to eat... I tell folks all the time that working is my hobby. The guys at work laugh at me all the time about how I work. They don't understand that this is how I was brought up. All the men on my dad's side of the family worked the same way. I always seem to get under other coworkers' skin about how I work. It does hurt me when I see folks that don't work as hard as me. Every time somebody works with me, they hate it. They say I work too hard and they can't keep up. That's all for now. Got to go to bed so I can go back to work. Can't wait.

Dec. 5, 2012: I had a great day of work. Got some orders done. We need to get more done. Time is not on my side. The holidays make it twice as hard to get orders done. I wish we were closer to being done than what we are. I need the guys to step up and get more built. They also need to understand they need to put their home life on hold till we get done. The company comes first around holidays. Customers want their stuff on time just like you would. If they don't get it on time they could not order any more. This is the big reason I work so hard every day to get them their orders. Plus I'd rather see a big smile on someone's face when we get the job done. It gives me that nice fuzzy feeling. Got to go. Write more stuff tomorrow.

I pity Erek working like this, but I understand and appreciate what he gets in return for what he gives up. I'm a teacher now, and he makes a lot more money than I do, but still not enough for what he sacrifices. My legs don't hurt and I can go to the bathroom anytime I want without feeling guilty about it. I know that however well his company is taking care of him, it can't be relied upon. Neither can the colleges that employ me. No company can.

I work like my father, just on different things. I teach, and put a lot of effort into it no one else can see. I know I won't be rewarded for teaching because these days nobody is rewarded for teaching. I write the way my father works on his projects. I cook the same way. I'm solitary about it. I improvise with what I have on hand. I recognize his ingenuity in me, and hope to do some justice to it in its new applications. I've tried to tell him how much I've realized we have in common, how I've inherited his operating system. I don't think he's convinced.

Posture of the Initiated Instructor

Stand where your instructors once stood. Figure out your own gestures and rhythms and intonations. Recall the first time you observed the blossoming mind of a student who trusted themselves to you—not when they only echoed you, but when they first took a tool you handed them and used it in their own way, to their own purpose. Make private metaphors for yourself out of hammers and axe handles and assisted wrenches. More clearly, now, notice what, across the work, remains the same. Start to lose your stupid romance for sweat labor, even as you retain respect for it. You no longer share what work you do, but you share the ways in which you do it. Try to tell your father that the two of you are much more alike than either of you realized. Come away pretty sure that he doesn't believe you. Keep knowing that anyway.

Posture of the Socially Aware

Assume a meditative pose when you take your shower. Remember that you used to take your shower at night because the work of your people and the scorching weather of their territory are such that you cannot go to bed carrying the filth of the day. As you wash away what has accumulated on you, consider that you must labor to contribute, to replenish what you consume, to compensate the world for the burden of your existence. Continue nodding in recognition of laborers, while any professional physical labor of your own recedes steadily into the past. Take care not to expect recognition in return. You avoided what they spend their lives doing. Settle for them thinking it is only admiration, since they won't be able to see themselves in you, since your hands are soft again. In them you won't witness who you used to be, only who you could have been.

I wonder when my children will take their showers, if I have children and if they grow up. I wonder what they work like, and why.

Posture of the Soft-handed Man

Feel your forearm, smooth now—the cross-hatched burnings long healed. Feel instead your guitar calluses and kitchen wounds— mostly cuts and burns. Consider the kitchen tools and tactics you've improvised. Consider the machines you built out of words. Consider physics, geometry, engineering, chemistry. Still enjoy splitting firewood because you only rarely get to do it. Long to move your mind and muscles in old, familiar ways, even when you live in apartments and there is no wood to split, no grass to cut, no wrenches to turn. Occasionally, gratefully, find furniture to fix, insulation to install, rust with which to contend.

Posture of the Stranger Among the Other Kinds of Faithful

Move from Alabama to Ithaca, New York. Release the pose of Driving-the-U-Haul and shift into the unfamiliar shape of Pedestrian-among-Pedestrians. Approach a random person and complain about any ailment. The first of the many panaceas you'll hear in reply—chiropractic, reflexology, acupuncture, gluten-free local organic non-GMO vegan diets, any medicine as long as it isn't "Western"—will likely be yoga. Notice that it's said as an obvious given. Don't assume there is no value or validity to any particular advice, but observe another pattern across seemingly incompatible things. Consider the tone. Consider that these remedies are described exactly as you've heard other simple miracle choices described: Go to church. Get to work. Let go. Mind your business. See that while the faith may be different, the faithfulness functions identically, at least among the loudest believers.

Reasonable people abound, silently, in all places. Astonish the Alabamian who complains of any ailment of body or mind by saying "I'm not going to tell you to go to church, or to simply work through it." Surprise the ailing Ithacan with, "I'm not going to tell you to do yoga or to go on an all-quinoa diet." Say to them both that whatever their ills, they are more complicated than that. Say that you will listen before claiming to know them, before deciding you are qualified to advise them. Then listen.

There were rare times in both places when I expected one kind of sermon or another, but I got empathy instead. For those I remain grateful. Work. Yoga. Religion. As magical medicines, we expect too much from them, we break ourselves with overdoses. We're so obsessed with cures for our ailments that we ignore their causes.

Final Posture of the Devotee

Assume a rest position. You decide what it looks like, though it probably involves an inclined hospice bed. Seek the realization that there is nearly nothing about which you can be truly certain. You can arrive here the easy way or the hard way—by watching others or by getting here yourself. Either way, carefully attend to both body and mind. See the lingering strength in your elderly grandfather's weary muscles, even as his shoulder gave in long ago from holding the heavy jack to the ceiling of the mine, even as what started as black lung evolves into a fatal tumor blocking a bile duct in his liver, even as the American labor in which he believed so strongly fails to reconstitute itself in the new globalized economy. Toward the end, he mutters little but "Greed done bout rurnt this country."

See your father's kidney stones—which worsen in the dehydration of shop work in Alabama summers. See the circulation problems in his legs from a genetic defect and a lifetime of squatting, kneeling, working in all kinds of poses but always on his feet when he wasn't on a tractor. See what the sun did to his skin. Feel the hardness of his hands from work and weather and time and chemicals. Recall the time when the strength of his own forearm was so great that what gave was not the pliers or the vise or the rusted-stuck object, but the tendon for which the strength of muscle and the stubbornness of rust were too powerful. See him in his last year before he quits his work at his own shop. Or at least it's what he hopes is his last year. Notice the degree of tilt in his recliner, where he spends more and more time these days.

I read of expert yogis in the West who've deteriorated their hips, destroyed their knees, worn away the cartilage and bone of their spine to the point of infirmity. And yet some still teach classes, still lead others to do likewise, though they must teach it lying down. I wonder if it's all of America that thinks we're not doing something well enough unless we do it until it kills us.

With the current work of my hands, I must seek exercise. Exercise is not merely avoidable; it actively avoids me. Grading papers is akin to sanding in its tedium, but it's apparently worse for the body. I recently read an article that questioned whether sitting would be my generation's smoking, the public health crisis of our time. I wonder if I'm killing myself while I'm writing this. Occupational hazards.

I wonder what will my own children be devoted to, or not, and why? What will my devotion to them look like? What will I have to wait for? What will I have to do while I'm waiting? What will they think of the work of their grandfathers and their fathers before them? Will they reject it? Will they long for it? Will they return to it? Would I want them to?

Keep working, whatever the work looks like. Maintain a low-grade anxiety about recliners and furniture that bends at similar angles. Halfheartedly avoid them. Find you can carry little with you except your sustaining suspicion of anything that promises to save you, that promises to save everybody.

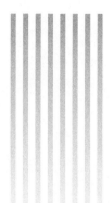

PART FOUR
LET GO

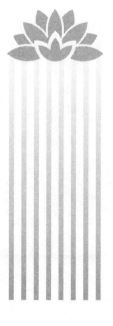

Gloria Muñoz

Corpse Pose

1.

In Corpse Pose on the wooden floor, every inhale buries you, the ebb and flow of it all engulfs you. Playing dead, and being cradled by the ground. A voice encourages you to *Relax, continue breathing, let go.* Palms are open and surrendering toward the ceiling; toes, fingers, and tongue are limp. You inhale, then exhale deeply through your nostrils. You are present.

2.

There are very few things I am masterfully good at. One of them is sleeping. I suppose I have been a very deep sleeper for a long time. Whenever I mention that I am tired at holiday gatherings, my family seizes the opportunity to remind me that I won the Best Sleeper Award in kindergarten. This has become a running joke in my family because it's my first academic achievement.

3.

No matter how many cups of coffee I've had, no matter how worried or excited or anxious or stressed I am in bed, I have no problem drifting off. And, to top that off, I am a still sleeper. That is to say, I wrap myself in my quilted blanket, pick a position, and stay in that position until I wake up. I don't snore. I don't wake up in the middle of the night. I don't get bothered by light or sound. Once I am asleep, I seem to be out cold. When we first started living together, my boyfriend, now husband, would wake up throughout the night and press his cheek against my back to make sure I was still breathing.

4.

My malaria pills were the only thing that ever kept me from sleeping in India. On my cot on the top floor of my host family's house, I lie awake wrapped in a white sheet. The room is dark, the walls are damp with humid air, the fan rattles from the ceiling, a stream of moonlight or lamplight runs across the floor. I am sweaty and covered in bug bites that run up and down my arms and legs. I've read and reread every book in my room. I have finished my Tamil homework and organized what I'd like my apartment to look like in the summer, what I'll eat for lunch from the market tomorrow, how I will convince my host mother that I am safe commuting on my bike, how I will describe each day here to my family when I get back. But I can't let my guard down, because she will come, the woman with the tattered black hair. She is old and missing a leg and covered in a layer of dust. She wears a ripped sari that once could have been white or lilac but is now as gray as her gums, to which she hold her fingertips, telling me *miss miss food miss food.* She'd come to my room every night to beg.

5.

My yoga instructor rubs lavender oil into my temples and scalp. My sweat comingles with essential oils. My mat is humid and it clings to my bare shoulders, arms, and calves; the small of my back is the only thing that retains its curve, a warm twilit sky, a rabbit's hole, a gravestone. After class my instructor tells me I've gotten better at Savasana, at being a corpse.

6.

While I lived in India, my friend Annie and I would meet at a tiny thatched-roof ashram midway between our host houses to practice yoga twice a week. At the end of every class we'd lie in meditation, in Savasana, for about twenty minutes. Perhaps it was the heat, or the lack of sleep, that made Savasana the time when I felt the most stillness in India. The sounds of traffic and temple speakers, the sensation of mosquitoes and ants and spiders creeping onto me, the snoring of old Indian men in the class—all ceased. Of course, these things were all still there. When I opened my eyes and came back from Corpse Pose, I was sure to find new bug bites, blaring car horns and speakers, and the old men stirring from their deep sleep, but, while I was in Savasana, the loud and irritating quality of these things vanished.

7.

My nephews are read to and sung to as they fall asleep each night, so they will be kept, so they will wake up. I remember the heavy fog between being awake and asleep as a child, the space where nonsense gibberish begs for one more story, line, embrace, song, one more moral ending. Children grow calm hearing their parents singing, *sleep, sleep, there's nothing to fear, it will be all right*—each withheld vowel, a tiny cry, pleading. Lullabies are meant to prepare people for dying.

8.

Doesn't it turn you on? Annie asked me once after a long time in Savasana. I associated lying on the dirt and meditating with many things, but not sex. *I think I had an orgasm, that time,* she continued, and then went into a rhapsody that went something like this: *It's a turn-on. You know, you are lying there, on the floor in tight yoga clothes, after a long and sweaty class, I mean really, you are sweating all over, with everything wide open, your legs, and your arms and palms and your "third eye"…*

9.

My metronomic bedtime ritual: In Spanish twice, in English once, as a child I prayed to Mary, to Jesus, to God. Santa María, Madre de Dios, ruega por nosotros, pecadores… Hallowed be your name… Padre nuestro, que estás en el cielo… Dios te salve, María, llena eres de gracia… Thy kingdom come, thy will be done… Ahora y en la hora de nuestra muerte… Now, and in the hour of our death… In the name of the father, the son, y El Espíritu Santo. Amen.

10.

With feet and knees flared and an unclenched jaw, we're lying on our backs, lips slightly parted, eyes mostly closed. This is the final resting pose. Incense burns notes of sandalwood and bergamot into the dampened studio floor. Lying faceup in a room full of people imitating corpses. The class breathes a collective reprieve—we live with death scratching at the backs of our hands.

Katherine Riegel

Why

I try to stay in my body during yoga class. I do. I try not to think of anything beyond the muscle, the stretch, the breath. But really I am anticipating the end of class, my favorite part, the payoff: Savasana.

Because sometimes I need to cry. I feel tears pushing at the back of my throat. I see an old woman hoist herself up from a chair and I think of my mother, gone these five years. I remember my nightmare, how this time I couldn't even remember the name of the boy I loved who lived over the hill from me in the Eden that was my childhood neighborhood. I need to cry but I can't, can't muster the self-pity that usually pushes me over the edge, can't get past the safeguards I've built over the years to hold hurt in. I want to close my eyes and loosen my mind.

The instructor tells me to arch my back like a cat. Sway my back. Arch again. Now lift my hips up to Downward Dog. I slowly walk my hands back toward my feet. I feel the blood push into my head, and think of my mother and grandmother, both diagnosed with glaucoma. The pressure isn't good for my eyes, but it's a basic yoga move. And I like dogs.

Because some books told me yoga and meditation were good for me. My favorite book admitted no one really knows why, but cited scientific studies about increases in the ability to focus, the ability to handle stress, positive effects on blood pressure and heart rate. Some books promise things like happiness, and those are the ones I don't trust. I like the ones that say there is no single right way to pose or meditate, you're not doing it wrong, some good will come of this but we're not promising anything. I don't know about my focus or blood pressure numbers. I haven't done studies on myself. But when I can't figure out what else to do, when I need *something* and whatever that need is feels aching and mysterious and hopeless, this is, at least, something to do.

Every time, no matter how frequently or infrequently I do yoga, my hamstrings scream. They start with the first pose and get louder and louder, working up from whimper to whine to cry to yell to constant keening. They don't remember being eight years old and doing the splits all the way down, how much I wanted to be like Nadia Comaneci. They only remember that I failed to complete a somersault in the air, landing hard on my ass enough times to knock the gymnastic dreams out of me.

Because sometimes during Savasana I begin to remember the rules I want to live by. For moments at a time I might remember and actually feel that I am living in the present and that worrying about invasive Cuban tree frogs or my upcoming dental appointment or when my car will break down is not, actually, required. If I have a mantra, it is *nonjudging, nonstriving.* During Savasana I might feel, very briefly, that my life is worthwhile *even when I'm not doing anything.*

At my gym, the instructor sometimes gives students the option of leaving after the stretches and poses and before Savasana. I watch them go, thinking, These are the same people who easily forgo dessert. I live for dessert. The poses are meat and potatoes and vegetables, the instructor's soothing voice flavoring the meal with reminders to breathe and half-truths about how well we're doing, how each of us is perfect. I need quiet and stillness to let that positive outlook seep in, to taste the sweetness.

Because it's not magic. I've had magic, in the form of certain kinds of pills, antianxiety and tiny and white and made of ground-up wishes sprinkled with glitter. I loved those pills. I knew immediately I could become addicted to them. If I have a craving greater than chocolate, it is sometimes for those little pills, which I used only once, during a period of a few months, and which—along with my sister and the love of several people and animals—saved my life. I don't trust magic, though. I don't want to live off those ground-up wishes. I want to want to live. Savasana brings me right up to the edge of sleep. It is awkward and a little silly, closing one's eyes while awake and pretending to be dead; I often feel my muscles vibrating like rubber bands in this quiet period. But I like that it's not magic. It's grounded in this world. It is not made of wishes but of space, space I need in which to imagine what I might do with my life.

The hard wood floor pressing into my shoulder blades through the thin yoga mat. The breathing in, and the space inside my chest; and the breathing out, and the space above and around me. The listening and not listening for the chime to indicate the end of class, time to open my eyes, go home. Suspension. Perhaps the chime will never come, and this space inside and around us all will expand to encompass the whole world, everything. Every time, there is possibility. That's what I come for.

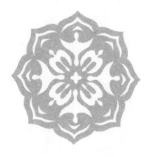

Emily Rapp

Being Seen

I will never be good at yoga. This was the recurring thought I had during my first yoga class in Austin, Texas, nearly ten years ago. That year I was finishing graduate school, writing my first book, and ending a marriage. A friend suggested yoga as a way to navigate this tricky stage that was both joyous and sad. I was also ready for an exercise routine that wasn't just about watching the clock tick down as the count for "calories burned" went up. I was ready for a change.

My first class was an Ashtanga series taught by a blond stick of a woman with a French accent who could do a full, unassisted backbend. I watched her body bend back like a wire, with ease and without breaking a sweat. During the class I followed her instructions to the best of my ability, which was a challenge given my artificial leg, but I managed to finish the class. When we had finished and were lying on our backs I continued to sweat and my muscles were already sore. I felt a sense of uneasy accomplishment, although we were told repeatedly that this was not the end result in yoga. As we sipped tea in the changing area outside the studio, I wasn't sure I'd ever return. This type of exercise required more concentration than just hopping on the treadmill and counting the minutes and steps. As a former anorexic, I was very committed to tangible yet unrealistic results: numbers on a scale, calorie counts recorded in a book.

I can't remember what made me "return to the mat," as they say. Perhaps it was the sweet and spicy tea served at the end of class, though I suspect it had more to do with the way I watched bodies differently after doing yoga. In other words, I stopped seeing bodies as fat or thin, disabled or normal, good or bad, at least for the length of the class. This was a great relief to me. As someone who starved herself for years as a way of compensating, I thought that, for one with an imperfect body, a body that couldn't be "fixed," yoga was a kind of exercise that eliminated any score keeping or ranking in terms of who was better or who was worse. These categories disappeared entirely; instead, we were asked to do what we could do in the moment. I had always wanted to be thin, I had always wanted two functional, long and lean legs, because I believed that would make me, in an illogical turn that only the neurotic can make, a good person. I wanted to be good, I wanted to be accepted, I wanted a place in the world. Yoga changed the relationship I have with my body by forcing me to understand that it was not a fixed entity to control but an embodied presence to be enjoyed. I found that some days I could balance, some days I could not. I found that I had more upper-body strength than I had counted on. I found that I stopped worrying about the way I looked doing a pose, and just found a way to do it. I stopped trying to be good.

One day, in the middle of practice, on a day when I was finding the poses particularly difficult, the teacher approached me and said, "You have a beautiful practice." I had always wanted to hear that I had a beautiful body, although I knew part of me would always resist that that could possibly be true. Disabled women are not models. Disabled women do not appear in magazines or movies. We're taught to hide our bodies, and some of us learn to do it well. I felt, in that moment of acknowledgment, *seen*. Not for looking a particular way or for conforming to some norm, but for simply being present in that room, in the moment, in that particular place, in that particular time.

True yoga isn't about being technically skilled, and it's never been about being good, as hard as it is to believe these statements. It's about being present, being alive, and for me, being truly seen. Now, instead of thinking *I will never be good at yoga,* I think *I love to do yoga.* A subtle change, but a transformative one.

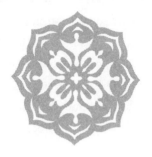

Dani Shapiro

On the All of It

I'm writing this in a crowded cafe in downtown Wilmington, North Carolina. My thirteen-year-old son is sitting across a round table from me. We're both clacking away on our laptops—he's ostensibly doing homework. He's drinking a vanilla steamer. Me, a cappuccino. It's loud here. Conversation, music, a blender making smoothies. Our suitcases are under the table, because we're being picked up in a few hours to be taken to the airport—on our way home after five days visiting my husband, who is directing his first film here.

How do we hold on to ourselves when life isn't routine—which is to say, most of the time? I am a creature of habit, quite possibly neurotically so. I eat the same thing for lunch every day, for instance

(Liberté Yogurt). I make my bed the minute I awake in the morning. I have certain requirements: solitude, silence, enough hours, caffeine. But for a while now, nothing has been routine. I've finished a book, and I'm nowhere near starting a new one. (I'm never near starting a new one until the day I do.) I've been writing a little of this, a little of that. My husband is away for months. My kid is in eighth grade, and we're looking at high schools. It's a particularly rich, completely nutty time.

In the midst of this, yesterday, someone (OK, a lady blow-drying my hair) asked me where I find inspiration. The question stopped me, for a moment, because I realized that I was very far from inspiration because the practices that allow me access to myself behind myself (to paraphrase Emily Dickinson) had fallen by the wayside. I hadn't packed my yoga mat on this trip. I had only managed to practice once. Meditation? As if. Reading? I had brought *Cloud Atlas* with me on the flight down, but had read *Vogue* instead.

"Everywhere," I answered the hair stylist. "I find inspiration everywhere, as long as my eyes are open."

Ah, but this is it—what it's all about—this openness. We writers (if I may generalize) are such sensitive creatures. I've heard it said that we're born with one less layer of skin than most people. Maintaining this openness—when in the midst of the noise, the crowds, life's dailiness, can be incredibly challenging. When I'm home and in my routine, I find it easier to be open because my routines support me. But it's a luxury, and unrealistic, to think that I can live that way all the time.

So I look around me. The boy, scribbling now in his math notebook. The woman behind the counter who also works in the local theatre. The smells and tastes. This unfamiliar town. I remind myself to breathe deeply, to fill my lungs, to stop *protecting* myself—from what? This noise, this pace, this tumult, right now, today, this is my life. If I am not present for it, if I'm simply getting through it until I'm finally back in my house on top of the hill with my bed made and my yoga mat unrolled, my favorite yogurt in the fridge, the silence and space and solitude I crave but can't always have—well, then. All sorts of gifts may pass me by.

Lately, when I attempt to sit down to meditate (notice the word attempt) I am almost instantly filled to the brim with feeling. This feeling isn't exactly bad, or exactly painful. It's characterized more by a kind of fullness that threatens to overflow. My throat constricts. My eyes well with tears. My heart pounds just a little bit harder, to let me know that it's there. Feeling. *Ready or not,* seems to be the beat of my heart. *Ready or not.*

I am writing this at my kitchen table. My family is still upstairs asleep. Even the dogs have left me alone. This is not the usual shape of things in my house. Usually I'm the last out of bed. But rain pounds on the rooftop—our little dog was up all night because he's terrified of storms—and so we all slept fitfully. As I look around my dark, solitary kitchen, I take it all in: The bowl of lemons on my kitchen table. The counter top covered with equipment—coffee maker, cappuccino machine, blender, toaster. A basket with every kind of vitamin known to man. Dried peppers from our garden. Envelopes with galleys of *Still Writing* waiting to go out in today's mail. Behind me, my son's tennis racket and a new Frisbee he just bought that apparently flies lower and faster and farther than any Frisbee ever before.

Also on my kitchen table, my well-worn book of Buddhist wisdom. It's old now. Its pages are wavy and stained, its spine all but fallen off. Today's quote is from Kalu Rinpoche: "From possession is born need. From non-attachment, satisfaction."

Oh, but it is hard to be unattached. Unattached to the people I love most in the world, sleeping upstairs. Unattached to the health of my body as I sit here writing. Unattached to the little books in those envelopes. Unattached to the home around me where I have raised my son. I glance upward at two pictures hanging on the wall. They were taken for a magazine five minutes ago—but wait, my son is small. My husband's hair is darker. I am younger. In one of them, Jacob sits on the kitchen counter and kisses me on the lips. It has been years since he's sat on the kitchen counter. Years since he's wanted to kiss his mother on the lips.

From non-attachment, satisfaction.

I'm always exhorting my writing students to do the work and then let go. To do the work, and understand that the rest—the rest is none of our business. I quote Martha Graham on making dance: "It is not your business to determine how good it is, nor how valuable it is, nor how it compares with other expressions." Graham goes on to write to her friend Agnes de Mille that it is only her business to keep it uniquely hers. She understood that our lives are as individual as snow-flakes. That we must, if we are artists—hell, if we are human beings—be focused only on the work, and letting go. The work, and letting go.

Ready or not, my heart continues to beat. *Ready or not.*

My son is going off to boarding school in September. My

husband has made the second massive career switch in his life—from foreign correspondent to screenwriter and now, to filmmaker. My writing life continues to transform in ways I could never have imagined. Everywhere I look, life is changing. Grace Paley once told my friend Amy Bloom that between the ages of fifty and eighty, it's not minutes, it's *seconds*.

And so, at my empty kitchen table, I take a deep breath, past the thickness in my throat. I let it all in—the all of it—the grief, sadness, joy, exhilaration, anxiety, fear, loss, and triumph of a lifetime. What other choice do I have? Upstairs, my family is stirring. Somewhere, someone is taking a shower. The dogs stretch and yawn.

Another precious day begins.

This morning I made my son breakfast, as I have every weekday morning since he was in kindergarten. I have a system. I take out the bread and cheese and lunch meats for his sandwich; scramble the eggs, toast the English muffin; pour the orange juice. I make myself a cappuccino while he eats at the kitchen counter. Then, I arrange his lunch box with military precision, learned over nine years of early morning sandwich making. The juice box. The organic fruit roll-up. The Entenmann's soft-baked chocolate chip cookies. Years ago, I used to tuck a note in with his lunch. Full of x's and o's. Wishing him a great day. I would draw a little mommy smiley-face. *I love you so so so so so so* much.

Today I made his early-morning breakfast and packed his school lunch for the last time.

He and my husband made their way down the stairs to the car, as I called after them: Drive carefully! Have a great day! See you later! My husband and I exchanged a glance. In that marital glance, there was all of it. The awareness this moment is one of tremendous change. That we are transitioning from one time in life to another. Just as the years of baby seats and plastic apparatus and bedtime stories gave way to tennis lessons and homework and class art projects, which in turn gave way to standardized tests and middle school dramas and team victories and defeats and boarding school applications, now we are entering a new phase, one which will reveal itself to us as we enter it. Our boy, our only boy, is going away to school next year. There is no road map.

After they left, in the quiet of my kitchen, I glanced down at the book of Buddhist wisdom that I keep on our table, open to today's offering. The wisdom of the day was from Pema Chödrön: "Thinking that we can find some lasting pleasure and avoid pain is what in Buddhism is called samsara, a hopeless cycle that goes round and round endlessly and causes us to suffer greatly."

And then I noticed the date. And realized that today is my mother's *yahrzeit*, the Hebrew anniversary of her death. She has been gone for ten years. I went into our dining room, where in the sideboard I keep a supply of yahrzeit candles. It is a measure of being at this stage of life—of having lost both of my parents—that I am always sure to have the candles around. (Our first year in rural Connecticut, I went out on the day before Yom Kippur to pick up a yahrzeit candle at the market, only to discover that I wasn't on the Upper West Side any more.)

Alone in the kitchen, having just sent my middle-schooler

off to his last day of eighth grade, full to the brim with the awareness that he will be going to high school four hours from home come September, I lit the candle for my mother and recited the Mourner's Kaddish. I thought of her with sorrow, with fondness, with confusion, with love. She and I had a complicated relationship. I wiped away my tears, and climbed the stairs to my office.

As I write these words, I am lying on my chaise longue surrounded by books. A former student's galley I intend to blurb, last week's *New Yorker*, a book for which I'm writing a literary appreciation, piles of galleys of *Still Writing*. My cappuccino has grown cold by my side. The dogs are curled up in their beds. The house is silent. Crows peck at the meadow outside my window. My boy is spending his last day at the only school he has ever known. My husband is at his office, digging in to work of his own. Downstairs, in the kitchen, a candle flickers.

This is it—all of it—a rich, deep, contemplative, paradoxical life—each hour full of the bitter and the sweet, the push and pull. Pleasure and pain in the same breath. To love is to risk. To love is to let go.

Lisa Knopp

Yoga through the Ages

1982

From Dandasana (Staff Pose), open the legs to form a ninety-degree angle," Petra said, as she led us into Upavistha Konasana (Seated Angle Pose). "Rotate your thighs toward the back of the room so that your kneecaps point to the ceiling." She paused. "Legs pressed into the floor." She paused again. "Feet flexed."

The five members of the class formed a row of seated right angles in front of a mirror-covered wall in the basement studio in Petra's house in Papillion, Nebraska. We were all in our twenties or early thirties. The two men were from the nearby Offut Air Force Base in Bellevue; we women drove to class from various parts of Omaha. Petra insisted that she be able to see our leg muscles and knees as we performed the asanas, so the men wore shorts while we woman wore shorts of leotards and tights, from which we'd cut the feet.

"Start walking your hands forward between your legs. Arms long. Bend from your hips instead of your waist. To maintain length in the front of your torso, lift the sternum," Petra said, her eyebrows lifting as her pitch rose. "Now stay here and check your alignment." I didn't want to stay here. I wanted to keep moving forward. But we were in for a substantial wait, since Petra was moving among us, making adjustments. She gently pulled me up by my shoulders. Once again, I'd gone farther into the posture than she wanted me to at that point.

I had taken my first yoga class in June of 1982, shortly after concluding my first year teaching English at a high school in Omaha. It had been a trying year, to say the least. I had taught two sections of American Literature to juniors and six sections of Grammar and Composition to sophomores. While I had a good background in American Literature, I knew next to nothing about grammar or how to teach writing. Too many days, I had gone home from a full day of work to a full evening of work: first learning the material that I had to present the next day; then figuring out how to teach it. With 135 students, I was grading all the time. None of the teacher education courses that I'd taken in college had prepared me to create a classroom environment that was at the same time orderly and disciplined, creative and responsive. Many days, I felt that I was engaged in a tug-of-war: me against a roomful of 15- and 16-year-olds.

Once the school year ended, I had time on my hands. I

enrolled in a couple of graduate classes at the local university and went in search of a physical discipline to bring balance into my sedentary life. When I was a child, I had been the misfit in physical education class who always lost the race, couldn't do a single chin-up, and on more than one occasion, was smacked in the face with the volleyball. Consequently, I wanted nothing to do with balls, teams, scores, and stopwatches. I supposed that I might enjoy something more individualized and less competitive, like one of the martial arts or yoga. I had watched a few reruns of "Lilias! Yoga and You" on PBS and knew that there was a difference between the way I felt after doing yoga stretches and breathing with Lilias Folan and after calisthenics in the "figure reducing" class I took as part of my physical education requirement at college: the latter was just exercise, but yoga created a glowing sense of spaciousness and well-being in my body and mind. I called the few yoga teachers listed in the Yellow Pages and chose Petra, who was easy to talk to and had a light, pleasing German accent.

"Keep the sternum lifted!" Petra exhorted, as she pulled up on an imaginary string connected to her breastbone. "And breathe." The six of us filled the room with the soft, sibilant hiss of ujjayi breathing. "Grab the big toes with your thumbs, index, and middle fingers. If you can't reach your toes, use a strap or grab your calves or ankles." One woman clasped her ankles; another woman and I hooked our fingers around our big toes. Because of their tight abductor and hamstring muscles, the men bent their knees and wrapped straps around their feet. I had been with the same group of people for week after week and knew what they could and couldn't do, and they knew the same about me. They knew that I had extraordinarily flexible hips joints and hamstrings but just a few seconds into Chaturanga Dandasana

(Staff Pose) or the arm balances, the very postures that Petra, a tiny, sinewy woman, and the two men excelled at, I started trembling and collapsed. I was far from balanced.

In yoga class, I was always anticipating the next step, always looking ahead. But Petra often asked us to stop, wait, and pay attention, which made me anxious, since I was far more comfortable with "doing" than "being." In my first few classes with Petra, she taught me how to stand and breathe—things that I thought I already did pretty well. In spite of my frustration with her insistence on mindful, diaphragmatic breathing and painstakingly precise alignment in Tadasana (Mountain Pose), I kept coming back.

I hadn't expected to be transformed by yoga. But during that first year of practice, I watched with surprise and delight as muscles that I hadn't known I had became firm and defined. Intuition told me that because of the centering effects of my yoga practice, I no longer needed the daily asthma medication I'd taken for years, so I gradually cut back until finally, I was free of the drug and my asthma was but an infrequent intruder. Several times, I read Paramahansa Yogananda's magical *Autobiography of a Yogi*, in which he teaches, through story and direct statement, that the end goal of yoga is samadhi, a state of union with God. And I read anything by or about B. K. S. Iyengar, the inspiration and discipline behind Petra's teachings. At the end of year one, I was attending a Thursday evening asana class and a Friday afternoon "jump class," where we flowed from one sweaty Surya Namaskar (Sun Salutation) to the next, and occasional weekend workshops on special topics—twists, backbends, inversions. Most important, I had committed myself to a daily, ninety-minute home practice followed by pranayama (breathing exercises) and dhyana (meditation). Yoga had quickly become the center of my life.

But there was much that I needed to surrender. I was evangelical in my efforts to teach the uninformed that the rigorous yoga I did was "real" yoga as compared to the soft, easy Lilias-style stretches that most people pictured when you said that you practiced yoga. And there was my ego. Because of my flexibility, I could easily hook a foot behind my head, rest both legs on the floor in splits, and practically bend in half in advanced backbends, poses that most people found challenging if not impossible. But Petra said that the students with their stiff joints, ligaments, muscles, and tendons knew more about the essence of yoga, which was releasing the inner pose through attention and surrender, than the super stretchy ones who could flop into any position but never went beyond the outer pose. Asana performance, she insisted, was the means not the end.

"If this is as far as you can go, stay here and breathe through the resistance," Petra advised. More waiting and sibilant breathing. "If you can go farther without collapsing the chest, rest your forehead on the floor." More waiting. "Now, rest your chin on the floor." Even more waiting. "And now your chest." This was the part of the posture I relished: the deep, delicious stretch of the inner thighs that resulted when I laid my head, chin and chest on the floor. Out of the corner of my eye, I could see that no one else had come this far.

June 1983, one year after I started yoga, Petra and I drove to Denver to take private lessons with two of her teachers, both of whom had studied with K. Pattabhi Jois and B. K. S. Iyengar. Somewhere during the long drive along the Platte River Valley and into the High Plains of eastern Colorado, Petra told me that after all these years of yoga study and practice, she was just beginning to catch glimpses of the freedom that Iyengar says is possible through yoga. I had no idea what she was talking about.

1992

Every morning, I did yoga, usually in sweat pants and a tee or sweat shirt in my living room with my two children nearby, *Sesame Street* on the television, and my then-husband working in his home office with NPR blaring. I'd jump through a handful of Sun Salutations, perform a few standing asanas, and then move to the floor for sitting postures and inversions. If I found a few minutes afterward for Savasana (Corpse Pose) or meditation, I often fell asleep.

I hadn't taken or taught a yoga class, worn a leotard, or practiced in front of a mirror in several years. I still read *Yoga Journal* but was more interested in the articles about "conscious living"—karma, shamanism, folk medicine, resurrecting the goddess, finding the sacred in the everyday, and Judith Lasater's wise columns about yoga philosophy—than those about performing asanas. Occasionally, I'd pick a few postures and follow Iyengar's instructions in *Light on Yoga* step by step, aware of how sloppy I'd become now that I was without a teacher and now that I rarely practiced in solitude. Even so, the yoga was still powerful. My time on the mat each morning helped me manage the demands of childrearing, a live-in sister-in-law, graduate classes, a teaching assistantship, an often stormy marriage, and the growing desire to write essays and books, but too little of the time required by such an endeavor.

Sometimes I looked into my future and wondered if life would always be this hectic. I read that in traditional Indian culture, a man attempted to structure his life according to the four *ashramas* or stages of spiritual life. The first stage is *bramacharya*, the student stage, in which one works closely with a spiritual teacher. For me, that was my period of study with Petra followed by all that I learned while teaching yoga at a community college. *Bramacharya* is followed by *grihastha*, the householder stage, in which one is primarily focused on fulfilling one's responsibilities toward family and society. I was squarely positioned within this stage and would be for many years to come. At around age fifty, one becomes *vanaprastha*, the hermit, who deepens his spiritual practice while lessening his connections with family and society. I supposed that when I turned fifty, my then twenty-two-year-old son would have finished college or military service and be starting his profession, whatever that might be; my then seventeen-year-old daughter would be preparing to leave home for college in a faraway part of the country; and I would be a tenured professor with many years of work ahead of me. I also supposed that I would either be divorced or married again. Would there be more time, then, for yoga classes and sustained meditation? According to the *ashrama* system, at about seventy-five, one becomes a *sannyasa*, a wandering renunciate or ascetic, who withdraws from worldly pursuits and channels his energies into his spiritual practice. While I had a dim picture of myself at fifty, I simply could not imagine myself at seventy-five, though certainly I'd still be practicing yoga. Nonetheless, I believed that this schema or road map would guide me through the different stages of life. Though developed for men, surely it could be adapted to the life of a woman living in North America at the turn of the millennium.

Those of us who were *grihastha* had little time and energy for a sustained practice of asana, pranayama, and meditation. But the *ashrama* system sets forth that as we householders earned money, cared for children, spouse, and parents, and performed our social duties, we could practice yoga while in the thick of it, by cultivating a loving relationship with God through acts of devotion (bhakti yoga) and by selflessly offering the fruits of our labors to God (karma yoga). Through these practices, we could be in the world yet not be overcome by it.

But overcome by the world was exactly how I felt. The idea that everything I did—from grading papers to cleaning the cat litter box—was for God, and therefore needed to be done with love and awareness, often eluded me. Even so, without yoga, I would have felt even more overwhelmed by the thousands of details involved in maintaining a home, family, and profession. The handful of asanas that I did each morning gave me a few minutes of peace and clarity before I got my son and myself ready for school, kissed my daughter and husband goodbye, dropped my son off at school, drove my sister-in-law and me to the university in time for our first classes, and then went to work earning my paycheck and my doctoral degree. Yoga worked for me.

The pose that I most looked forward to performing each morning was Adho Mukha Svanasana (Downward-Facing Dog Pose). But rarely did I practice it without distraction or hold the pose for as long as I wanted. As I moved into Downward Dog, I lengthened my spine and hamstrings and dropped my head toward the floor. "I do that," my daughter said as she stuck her diapered bottom into the air and looked at me from between her legs. "Peek-a-boo!" I said. My son appeared in the doorway, still in his pajamas. "I don't have anything to wear," he said. "My clothes are in the dryer and they're wet."

"I'll be there in one minute," I said. I dropped my heels into the floor, lifted my buttocks toward the ceiling, and breathed evenly and expansively, as the knots and tangles in my body-mind loosened. For a few moments, I was positioned in the calm eye of the storm.

2002

Drenching upper-body sweats often awakened me in the middle of the night. By the time I blotted myself dry with a towel and changed clothes, I was awake and my mind racing—my father's cancer, my teenage son's rebellion, my daughter's demanding extracurricular schedule, squabbles with my ex-husband, work and bills, plans and speculations. How could I do all that I expected of myself during the day if I was wide awake at 3:00 a.m.?

On one of those still dark, bleary-eyed mornings, instead of drinking enough black tea that I was buzzed on caffeine and then getting to work on my writing or on student manuscripts, I slipped a video into the VCR and I followed Richard Freeman through a long series of Sun Salutations. Arching, bending, pushing, folding, twisting, folding, pushing, bending. The sequence created heat in my muscles and settled my mind inward. When the tape was finished, I went back to bed and fell into a deep, silky sleep. When I awakened a few hours later, I was rested and grateful. Thereafter, if I awakened too early, I simply unrolled my sticky mat and went to work. I no longer feared the challenges of midlife and the insomnia, night sweats, and dark, heavy moods of perimenopause.

During my forties, I was particularly drawn to the balancing postures, such as Virabhdrasana III (Warrior III Pose), Bakasana (Crane Pose), Natarajarasana (Lord of the Dance Pose), and Ardha Chandrasana (Half Moon Pose). The latter was particularly gratifying. From Utthita Trikonasana (Extended Triangle Pose), I'd bend my right leg and place my right palm about a foot ahead of my right foot. As I shifted my weight onto my right hand and foot, I let my left leg float up. Once I straightened both of my legs and my right arm, my head, torso, leg, and foot formed a beautiful diagonal line suspended above the earth. Then I'd rotate my rib cage, opening my chest to the heavens. What I loved about Ardha Chandrasana is that the balance has to be renewed moment by moment, by spreading the toes, by pulling energy up the front thigh muscles, by gazing at a steadying point on the wall, by checking my alignment, by breathing. Otherwise, I'd wobble or topple. As with yoga, so with life. If I maintained a firm grounding and renewed my balance moment by moment, I was steady and serene.

Yoga taught me humility and perspective. At midlife, standing on my head or hooking my feet behind my head were no longer part of my practice, since there was no way that I could warm up enough to avoid getting a crick in my neck or back while practicing those asanas. Yet I was holding my own in most other postures. I found solace in the fact that the asanas would keep me strong and supple as I aged and that yoga was teaching me how to remain focused on the here and now instead of lost in regrets about the past (If only I had...) and anxiety over the future (Would I be healthy? Would I have enough money? Would I have enough people to love and to be loved by?). At this stage in my life, my yoga practice was far less concerned with rigidly forcing my asanas to resemble those performed by the twenty-something fashion model adepts featured in *Yoga Journal* than with being soft and open, firm and balanced, precise and playful, and above all, mindful. When I performed the postures with this attitude in mind, I could remain present and detached as waves of fear, joy, craving, resistance, judgmentalness, frustration, and pride washed over me. Yoga worked for me.

Once my children left home, my son in 2005 and my daughter in 2008, and I was no longer as consumed with the duties of the householder, I was free to begin transitioning into the hermit stage. Yet that wasn't what I was being called to. Even though my children were living under other roofs, I still had plenty of mothering ahead of me, since they needed my love, money, advice, and companionship. And, too, I was wild to connect more deeply with people beyond my job at the university and activities once related to my children. Deep into midlife, the schema that I was most drawn to wasn't that of the *ashramas* but that of the three archetypal faces of the feminine: maiden, matron, and crone, symbolized, respectively, by the waxing, full, and waning phases of the moon. Deep into midlife, I was posed on the cusp between mother and crone.

The manifestation in me of the mother archetype was one that I had both embraced, since I loved having given life to and nurturing my children, and sometimes resisted, since I found the demands of mothering, or rather single parenting, to be unrelenting and at times depleting. But there was nothing about the crone, who is usually presented as a wrinkled, shrunken, withered, witchlike old woman awaiting her own death, that attracted me until I read Barbara Walker's *The Crone: Woman of Age, Wisdom, and Power.* Walker portrays the crone as a "wise, willful, wolfish" woman, whose wrinkles are "badges of honor," and who possesses the wisdom, creativity, vitality, and experience that our society so badly needs. This was an aspect of the goddess that I was willing to grow into as I allowed my expression of the mother archetype to diminish.

When I performed Half Moon, I did so slowly, so that I embodied the unhurried and constant movement of the waxing and waning moon. Though I loved holding this asana, it was the transition between the poses that was teaching me how to live at this point. I moved from Tadasana into Utthita Trikonasana, forming triangles with my torso and limbs. As I held the posture, my body, breath, and mind became open and bright. As I tipped from Triangle into Half Moon, I was mindful of the wisp of sadness I felt as I let go of one beloved pose and the anticipation I felt as I moved into the next in the sequence. Once I was positioned in Half Moon, I savored the movement of energy around the bottom of my feet and up and down my legs, spine, and arms. Then, ever so slowly, I let go of my beautiful Ardha Chandrasana and returned to Trikonasana and then to where I began, in Tadasana. I turned and faced the other side and started the cycle anew.

2012

Many times each day, no matter what I was doing—washing dishes, practicing yoga, hanging out with friends, gardening, teaching, or writing—so much sticky phlegm rose in my throat that I felt gurgly. Coughing didn't help, though aggressively and repeatedly clearing my throat might bring brief relief. On several occasions, the mucus lodged in my trachea and I stopped breathing. If this happened in the presence of others, someone pounded on my back or shook me until the obstruction broke loose. If this happened when I was alone, only good luck and my panicky movements would apparently clear the blockage. But would this work every time?

Fear of suffocation led me to consult with my doctor. I suspected that an allergy was causing the phlegm. If I knew what the allergen was, I'd avoid it. But my doctor said that my symptoms were not caused by an allergic reaction. Gastroesophageal reflux disease (GERD), in which the contents of the stomach back up into the esophagus, was the culprit. The mucus that sometimes took my breath away was my body's attempt to protect the esophagus from irritation. Since the delicate lining of the esophagus can't tolerate gastric acid the way the stomach can, prolonged exposure can cause bleeding ulcers, inflammation, and scarring of the esophageal lining, which make breathing and swallowing difficult. Erosion of the lining is of particular concern, since it can lead to Barrett's esophagus, a condition in which the normal cell type that lines the lower part of the esophagus is replaced by intestinal cells. People with Barrett's are at a higher risk than those without it of developing esophageal cancer, one of the deadliest cancers.

A gastrointestinal specialist performed an endoscopy of my upper GI tract, which revealed that my lower esophageal sphincter (LES), that ring of muscle between the lower esophagus and the stomach, was weak. Most people with this problem find relief by taking a proton pump inhibitor (PPI), a class of drugs that stop the production of gastric acid. Because I couldn't tolerate the side effects of the several PPIs that I tried, my doctor suggested that I might be a good candidate for Nissen fundoplication, a procedure in which a surgeon strengthens the LES by wrapping the fundus, the upper curve of the stomach, around the valve and sewing it into place. From my research, I knew that this was a controversial surgery with side effects, such as the inability to burp or vomit, that seemed as harmful to me as those associated with GERD. Surgery, I decided, would be my last resort.

In the meantime, I took matters into my own hands. I tried several natural remedies: bromelain, a strongly neutralizing enzyme found in fresh pineapple; raw, organic apple cider vinegar, which hastens the digestion of fats; wild marshmallow root, which has slippery, coating properties; sodium alginic acid, a seaweed extract, which forms a viscous barrier between the gastric contents of the stomach and the esophagus. I adopted a low acid, high alkaline diet, which called for the elimination of most grains, fats, sugars, and animal products. Though I'd stopped eating meat decades ago, I sorely missed ice cream and yogurt. I worked with two practitioners of traditional Chinese medicine, one of whom said that my problem was "rebellious chi," since my vital energy wanted to go up instead of down. In talk therapy, I explored the metaphorical nature of fire in the belly, blockage in the throat, and a rebellious vital energy. Some of these efforts helped a little. But none helped very much.

At the same time, I altered the way I did almost everything so that my esophagus was always higher than my stomach. I jacked up the head of my bed and slept on a slope. I ate smaller and more frequent meals, so my stomach was never full. I ate nothing after 6:00 p.m.; drank nothing after 8:00 p.m. I continued to eat the curries and chilies that I love, since spicy foods created no more distress than bland ones. But because wheat had long upset my digestive tract, I adopted a gluten-free diet. I stopped leaping up stairs, bending over to pull weeds, running, dancing, or jumping with joy, since these movements could cause acid to rise in my esophagus. I no longer wore clothes with snug waistbands, since they put pressure on my stomach.

This was easy. Because of the dietary changes, I quickly shed over twenty pounds from my small frame. I hadn't weighed so little since middle school. But I wasn't happy. The lifestyle changes I'd made had little effect on the problem and left me feeling half starved and straightjacketed by restrictions. The more I tried to create balance in my digestive tract, the more out of balance my life became.

The greatest sacrifice was that I stopped practicing any asana that put my esophagus lower than or level with my stomach, which is most of them. No more luscious forward bends or inversions, since they allowed the contents of my stomach to slosh into my esophagus. No more open-hearted twists or backbends, since they pushed the stomach contents upward. No more flat-on-the-floor Savasana, though my yoga teacher did devise a way in which I could relax while remaining upright by reclining against bolsters propped against the wall. What I was left with was a handful of safe postures and a broken heart.

Some postures that I never enjoyed performing before, Virabhadrasana II (Warrior II pose), Vrksasana (Tree Pose), Utthita Hasta Padangusthasana (Extended Hand to Big Toe Pose), Hanumasana (splits), and those that I considered to be easy, beginner poses like Dandasana (Staff Pose) and Gomukhasana (Cow-Faced Pose), were precious to me simply because I could do them. But as the stubborn, strangling phlegm rose in my throat, I wondered if the day would come when I wouldn't be able to do a single asana. Is this what three decades of yoga and all those big and little lessons it had provided me about the grace, essence, and power of surrender had been preparing me for: to let go of my asana practice?

Most mornings, my yoga practice consisted of standing postures followed by Baddha Konasana (Bound Angle Pose), a posture that I had rarely practiced since it seemed to demand so little of me. As I sat on the floor with the soles of my feet pressed together, I ached to do Downward Dog or a deep twist. Yet Baddha Konasana offered everything I needed: the opportunity to leave my thinking mind behind and to be present in the here and now; to let go of my fears and desires; to be grateful for what I had; to see every posture as a prayer and my body as a living sacrifice. Baddha Konasana quickly became the crown jewel of my pared-down practice.

Despite these radical changes and my doctor's ongoing efforts to find a medication that I could tolerate, thick phlegm continued to clog my throat and steal my peace. Two doctors, one a specialist, had diagnosed my ailment as GERD, and I believed them. But I also believed that there was more to my condition than just that. I referred myself to the University of Nebraska Medical Center, where tests revealed that, much to my surprise, I was refluxing very little. The cause of my throat and breathing problems was achlasia (Greek for "failure to relax"), which refers to the inability of the LES valve to open and let food pass into the stomach, a diagnosis that seemed to conflict with the results of the endoscopy, which said that that valve was too relaxed. Achlasia can cause swallowing difficulties, chest pain, regurgitation, coughing, and, if food gets into the lungs, breathing problems. According to the Merck Manual, achlasia is caused by a malfunction of the nerves that control the rhythmic contractions of the esophagus. While the cause of the malfunction isn't known, it's clear that stress and anxiety worsen the symptoms.

The GI professor at the medical center recommended a calcium channel blocker or an antianxiety drug to relax the smooth muscles of my esophagus. If that didn't solve the problem, he said that he could stretch my esophagus with a balloon. I was relieved by the diagnosis, yet concerned by the treatments that he was recommending. If my condition was due, at least in part, to a "failure to relax," the right prescription was an even deeper and more committed yoga practice. If yoga couldn't heal me or mitigate my symptoms, then I'd try pills and procedures.

While I was troubled and at times angry, even, that I had lived with a wrong and expensive diagnosis for over a year and that I'd suffered in ways I shouldn't have had to, and though I was deeply unsettled by the fact that I had been asked to consider a surgery that might not have alleviated my symptoms and that, even worse, might have created others that were just as dangerous, my joy and relief were greater. I also felt empowered by the fact that I had listened to my intuition and sought a third opinion.

The effect of the new diagnosis had an immediate effect on my condition. As I walked from the GI doctor's office to the parking ramp, I felt light and free of the burden of a wrong diagnosis and questionable treatments. As soon as I arrived at the stall where I'd left my car, I gathered and quieted myself in Tadasana. From there, I moved into Utthita Trikonasana and from there into Parivrtta Trikonasana (Revolved Triangle Pose), holding the latter a generous amount of time on each side. Never before had I enjoyed the exquisite stretch and torsion of my torso as much as I did in that light and free moment in a dark and oil-stained hospital parking ramp. That day, I went off all prescribed drugs and began reducing my use of antacids and other neutralizing agents. Because I'd grown to appreciate smaller and more frequent meals and sleeping with my head slightly elevated, I continued with those practices.

Even though I'm still not able to do asanas that put my esophagus lower than my stomach, since the pressure they create triggers my achlasia, I have incorporated a wider range of postures back into my practice. And I've used the symptoms of my condition as the launching point for an even deeper yoga, for an even more refined awareness of what I am experiencing in the eternal now, and as a way to open myself to possibilities that I can't imagine.

Each morning, as I move through standing and floor postures, I give myself to yoga, skin to soul. The knots and stresses dissipate, and the voices in my head that rattle on about emails, deadlines, workplace and national politics, and all the big and little ways that I've wronged myself and others and they me, become softer, less insistent. Sometimes, they even stop. Finally, I'm ready for Baddha Konasana. I sit on the floor and press the soles of my feet together and lift my spine. With eyes softly gazing at the floor just beyond my feet, I allow my hips to release, my stomach to soften, my shoulders to drop, and my chest and throat to open. I observe the air entering my nostrils, filling my lungs and leaving again, like the predictable, rhythmic movements of ocean tides or migrating sandhill cranes or the stages of the moon. I observe the stretch in my knees, thighs, groin, and the softening and opening of my esophagus.

Sitting in my morning prayer pose, I am open, serene, receptive, and attentive. B. K. S. Iyengar says that the aim or final destination of yoga is "freedom and beatitude." In these moments of centered, uncluttered awareness, I catch glimpses of this.

About the Authors

CLAIRE DEDERER's national best-seller *Poser: My Life in 23 Yoga Poses* (Picador) has been translated into eleven languages. Dederer is a longtime contributor to the *New York Times*, and her articles have appeared in *Vogue*, *Real Simple*, the *Nation*, *Yoga Journal*, on Slate and Salon, and in newspapers across the country.

SONYA HUBER is the author of two books of creative nonfiction, *Cover Me: A Health Insurance Memoir*, finalist for the ForeWord Book of the Year, and *Opa Nobody* (University of Nebraska Press), shortlisted for the Saroyan Prize. She has also written a textbook, *The Backwards Research Guide for Writers: Using Your Life for Reflection, Connection, and Inspiration*. Her work has been published in the *New York Times*, *Creative Nonfiction*, *Brevity*, *Fourth Genre*, the *Chronicle of Higher Education*, and the *Washington Post Magazine*. She teaches in the Department of English at Fairfield University and in the Fairfield Low-Residency MFA Program.

ELIZABETH KADETSKY is the author of the memoir *First There Is a Mountain* (Little, Brown) and, forthcoming, the story collection

The Poison That Purifies You (C&R Press) and a novella, *On the Island at the Center of the Center of the World* (Nouvella Books). Her fiction has been included in the Pushcart Prize collections, Best New American Voices, and the Best American Short Stories notable citations, and her personal essays have appeared in the *New York Times*, *Antioch Review*, and elsewhere. She is assistant professor of creative writing at Penn State, and can be found at elizabethkadetsky.com

LISA KNOPP is the author of five books of creative nonfiction. Her most recent, *What the River Carries: Encounters with the Mississippi, Missouri, and Platte* (University of Missouri Press), was the winner of the 2013 Nebraska Book Award for nonfiction/essay. Currently, she's working on a collection titled *Like Salt or Love: Essays on Leaving Home*, which will include "Yoga through the Ages." Knopp is a professor of English at the University of Nebraska–Omaha, where she teaches courses in creative nonfiction. She lives in Lincoln. Her website is lisaknopp.com.

BRENDA MILLER is the author of four essay collections: *Altered Fruit* (SheBooks), *Listening Against the Stone* (Skinner House Books), *Blessing of the Animals* (Eastern Washington University Press), and *Season of the Body* (Sarabande Books). She has also co-authored *Tell It Slant: Creating, Refining and Publishing Creative Nonfiction* (McGraw Hill) and *The Pen and The Bell: Mindful Writing in a Busy World* (Skinner House Books). Her work has received six Pushcart Prizes. She is a Professor of English at Western Washington University and serves as editor in chief of the *Bellingham Review*. Her website is www.brendamillerwriter.com.

AMY MONTICELLO's work has appeared in places such as Salon, *Brevity*, and the Nervous Breakdown, and was listed as notable in Best American Essays 2013. She is currently a visiting assistant professor at the University of Wisconsin–Eau Claire. She lives with her husband and daughter in Eau Claire, Wisconsin.

DINTY W. MOORE is the author of *The Mindful Writer: Noble Truths of the Writing Life* (Wisdom Publications), as well as the memoir *Between Panic & Desire* (Bison Books), winner of the Grub Street Nonfiction Book Prize in 2009. Moore has published essays and stories in the *Southern Review*, the *Georgia Review*, *Harper's*, the *New York Times Sunday Magazine*, the *Philadelphia Inquirer Magazine*, *Iron Horse Literary Review*, and the *Normal School*, among numerous other venues. A professor of nonfiction writing at Ohio University, Moore lives in Athens, Ohio, where he grows heirloom tomatoes and edible dandelions.

SUZANNE MORRISON is the author of *Yoga Bitch* (Random House/Three Rivers Press), which was a Crosscut Best Northwest Book of 2011 and has been translated into six languages. A recipient of 4Culture and Artist Trust grants, Suzanne is at work on a new memoir, *Your Own Personal Alcatraz*, about an early romantic entrapment on an island near Seattle. Her fiction and essays have appeared or are forthcoming in *Litro*, *Salt Hill*, Printers Row at the *Chicago Tribune*, the Huffington Post, *Crosscut*, and elsewhere. You can find Suzanne at her blog, suzannemorrison.blogspot.com.

GLORIA MUÑOZ holds a BA from Sarah Lawrence and an MFA from the University of South Florida. She has been honored by the

Estelle J. Zbar Poetry Prize, the Bettye Newman Poetry Award, the New York Summer Writer's Institute Fellowship, and the Think Small to Think Big Artist Grant. Her work has appeared in print and online publications including *Acentos Review*, *Dark Phrases*, the *Brooklyn Review*, the *Sarah Lawrence Review*, and, most recently, the *Best New Poets Anthology*. When not writing, teaching, and translating, Gloria teaches yoga and enjoys walking with Frida, her bearded beagle.

ADRIANA PÁRAMO is a cultural anthropologist, writer, and women's rights advocate. She is the author of two nonfiction books: *Looking for Esperanza* (Benu Press) and *My Mother's Funeral* (Caven-Kerry Press). Her work has won numerous awards and honors, has been nominated for multiple Pushcart Prizes, and has been noted in The Best American Essays of 2012 and 2013. She is currently working on a book about modern slavery in the Middle East. Páramo provides individual mentoring to inmates in the USA, and teaches zumba, Latin dances, and Spanish in Qatar.

NEAL POLLACK is the author of several bestselling books of fiction and nonfiction, including *Alternadad* (Random House), *Stretch: The Unlikely Making of a Yoga Dude* (Harper Perennial), and *Downward-Facing Death* (Thomas & Mercer). He has worked as a columnist for *McSweeney's*, *Vanity Fair*, *GQ*, Nerve.com, and the Faster Times.

EMILY RAPP is the author of *Still Point of the Turning World* (Penguin Press) and *Poster Child: A Memoir* (Bloomsbury). A former Fulbright scholarship recipient, she has received recognition for her work from the *Atlantic*, *StoryQuarterly*, and elsewhere. Her work has appeared in the *Los Angeles Times*, Salon, the *Sun*, and many other publications. Emily has taught writing in the MFA program at Antioch University–Los Angeles, The Taos Writers' Workshop, University of California–Palm Desert, and the Gotham Writers' Workshops. She is currently professor of creative writing and literature at the Santa Fe University of Art & Design.

KATHERINE RIEGEL is the author of two books of poetry, *What the Mouth Was Made For* and *Castaway* (FutureCycle Press), and a book about mindfulness and self-empowerment, *The Manifesto*. Her poems and essays have appeared in a variety of journals, including *Brevity*, *Crazyhorse*, and the Rumpus. She is co-founder and poetry editor for Sweet: A Literary Confection. Visit her at katherineriegel.com.

DANI SHAPIRO is the bestselling author of the memoirs *Devotion* and *Slow Motion* (Harper Perennial), and five novels, including *Black & White* and *Family History* (Anchor). Her work has appeared in the *New Yorker*, *Granta*, *Tin House*, *Elle*, the *New York Times Book Review*, and the *Los Angeles Times*. She has taught in the writing programs at Columbia, NYU, The New School, and Wesleyan University. Shapiro is co-founder of the Sirenland Writers Conference in Positano, Italy, and she is a contributing editor at *Travel + Leisure*. She lives with her family in Litchfield County, Connecticut. Her new book is *Still Writing: The Perils and Pleasures of a Creative Life* (Atlantic Monthly Press).

ALAN SHAW is a graduate of the MFA program at The University of South Florida. He is currently lobbing his memoir, *Ex-Mormon/*

Ex-Con—about being raised in the Mormon Church and the years he later spent in a Florida state prison—at every agent in every town. He teaches for USF's Honors College, where he also coaches the university's debate teams. Most days he makes excuses for the behavior of his ridiculously small dog. His work has appeared in Sweet: a Literary Confection, *Scissors and Spackle*, and *Spry* Literary Journal.

CHERYL STRAYED is the author of #1 *New York Times* bestseller *Wild,* the *New York Times* bestseller *Tiny Beautiful Things,* and the novel *Torch. Wild* was chosen by Oprah Winfrey as her first selection for Oprah's Book Club 2.0. The movie adaptation of *Wild* will be released by Fox Searchlight in December 2014. The film is directed by Jean-Marc Vallée and stars Reese Witherspoon, with a screenplay by Nick Hornby. Strayed holds an MFA in fiction writing from Syracuse University and a bachelor's degree from the University of Minnesota. She lives in Portland, Oregon, with her husband and their two children.

IRA SUKRUNGRUANG is a Thai American writer, teacher, and disc golf extraordinaire. He co-edited, with his good friend Donna Jarrell, *What Are You Looking At? The First Fat Fiction Anthology* and *Scoot Over, Skinny: The Fat Nonfiction Anthology* (Mariner Books). He is the author of a memoir, *Talk Thai: The Adventures of Buddhist Boy* (University of Missouri Press), and the poetry collection *In Thailand It Is Night* (University of Tampa Press). Currently he edits the Clever Title and Sweet: A Literary Confection. He teaches in the MFA program at the University of South Florida.

JASON TUCKER received an MFA from Ohio State University and currently teaches writing at the University of Wisconsin–Eau Claire. His essays have appeared in the *Southeast Review, River Teeth, Cream City Review*, the *Common, Sweet*, and *Waccamaw*.

About the Editor

 A New Yorker turned Floridian, **MELISSA CARROLL** is a writer, yoga teacher, and creative writing instructor at the University of Tampa. She is the author of *The Karma Machine* (YellowJacket Press), which received the Peter Meinke Award, and her work has appeared in the *Waterhouse Review, Creative Loafing,* the *Literary Bohemian, Poetry Quarterly,* and elsewhere. Melissa received her MFA from the University of South Florida. She was a National Park Service writer-in-residence in Arizona. Melissa discovered yoga and Reiki in 2006, and quickly realized the profound transformation these paths would have on her life. She currently teaches more than 250 students at the largest weekly yoga class in Florida, assists in the Yoga Loft's teacher training program, and leads workshops and retreats all over the world. Her classes are mindful, playful, and designed to help others discover inner peace. Visit her at melissacarrollyoga.com.

Photograph by Gordon Tarpley.

To Our Readers

Viva Editions publishes books that inform, enlighten, and entertain. We do our best to bring you, the reader, quality books that celebrate life, inspire the mind, revive the spirit, and enhance lives all around. Our authors are practical visionaries: people who offer deep wisdom in a hopeful and helpful manner. Viva was launched with an attitude of growth and we want to spread our joy and offer our support and advice where we can to help you live the Viva way: vivaciously!

We're grateful for all our readers and want to keep bringing you books for inspired living. We invite you to write to us with your comments and suggestions, and what you'd like to see more of. You can also sign up for our online newsletter to learn about new titles, author events, and special offers.

Viva Editions
2246 Sixth St.
Berkeley, CA 94710
www.vivaeditions.com
(800) 780-2279
Follow us on Twitter @vivaeditions
Friend/fan us on Facebook